New Frontiers in Men's Sexual Health

NEW FRONTIERS IN MEN'S SEXUAL HEALTH

Understanding Erectile Dysfunction and the Revolutionary New Treatments

K. Anthony Hanash, M.D.

Sex, Love, and Psychology
Judy Kuriansky, Series Editor

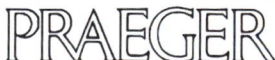

Westport, Connecticut
London

Library of Congress Cataloging-in-Publication Data

Hanash, Kamal Anthony.
  New frontiers in men's sexual health : understanding erectile dysfunction
and the revolutionary new treatments / K. Anthony Hanash.
      p. cm. — (Sex, love, and psychology, ISSN 1554–222X)
  Includes bibliographical references and index.
  ISBN 978–0–313–36263–7 (alk. paper)
  1. Impotence. I. Title. II. Series.
  [DNLM: 1. Erectile Dysfunction. WJ 709 H233n 2008]
  RC889.H253   2008
  616.6'92—dc22   2008026226

British Library Cataloguing in Publication Data is available.

Library of Congress Catalog Card Number: 2008026226
ISBN: 978–0–313–36263–7
ISSN: 1554–222X

First published in 2008

Praeger Publishers, 88 Post Road West, Westport, CT 06881
An imprint of Greenwood Publishing Group, Inc.
www.praeger.com

Printed in the United States of America

The paper used in this book complies with the
Permanent Paper Standard issued by the National
Information Standards Organization (Z39.48–1984).

10 9 8 7 6 5 4 3 2 1

My wife, France, and children, Tony, Patrick, Alain, and Carla, whose patience and encouragement made this book possible.

CONTENTS

FOREWORD

When I was hosting my radio call-in advice show every night for years, all topics were welcome. But as soon as one man called up about a problem with his sexual functioning, the phone lines were flooded with similar calls from worried males, with the result that I could spend the entire rest of the night talking about men's sexuality. The most common calls were from guys who were fearful that they were too small—when in fact their penis size was within normal range—and from guys worried about not lasting long enough, or having a hard time getting hard.

The age of men talking openly about their sexual problems has exploded. The good news is that—finally—men are not hiding in shame, thinking they don't measure up to a macho male societal image. But the open talk led to a shock—that so many men were suffering. Fortunately, over the years, more help has become available for every man's complaint.

In this book, *New Frontiers in Men's Sexual Health: Understanding Erectile Dysfunction and the Revolutionary New Treatments*, Dr. K. Anthony Hanash brings us up to date with all the complaints men have, and even better, with all the latest hope for solutions. A urologist, Hanash has professional credentials and 35 years of experience. In this book he backs up everything he addresses with the most solid, scientific, and up-to-date scientific research. In these pages, we find out about all that can go wrong for men, their partners, and also how to fix it.

Even I, who have been in the field of sexuality for as long, was rapt while reading these pages. Like a murder mystery, there were parts I couldn't put down, unraveling the medical and psychological mysteries of a man's sexual functioning and what can be done to solve the predominant complaints of size, desire, or performance. What Dr. Hanash gives us in these pages is a thorough review of the literature and scientific knowledge about male sexual functioning, in clear-enough language so we can truly understand the answers to pressing questions like "Is there a bone in the penis?" Or "Does anything really work to make the penis longer?" All this is then put into context of the man in his relationship, as partners are affected by any problem the man suffers.

Most compelling is the promise of the book's title—*New Frontiers in Sexual Health: Understanding Erectile Dysfunction and the Revolutionary New Treatments*—that we would discover in these pages revolutionary new treatments for male sexual problems. And indeed we do. Any health professional, and any man or woman, will be compelled by the exploration of the new frontiers presented here. Hanash keeps the reader amazed as he explores "Is sexual desire in the genes?" and as he describes experimental treatments and new products under study to treat male sexual problems. Some are intended for other purposes, like calcitonin, nitroglycerine, and minoxidil (for hair growth). Others are names of compounds the average person hardly recognizes now—like a PT-141 inhaler, or "recombinant erythropoietin" (a protein which stimulates the production of red blood cells)—but that may appear on the nightly news tomorrow as the next new hope,

In this book, Dr. Hanash has taken his extensive and intensive knowledge and made it understandable. In that, he has reached the goal he set for himself—to take a complex subject and make it simple enough for everyone to comprehend.

Dr. Judy Kuriasky
Series Editor

PREFACE

It is better to light a candle than to curse the dark.

Chinese proverb

The word *impotence* is derived from the Latin *impotentia*, or "lack of power." It has hounded men since the beginning of time. Impotence has triggered wars, lost kingdoms, tarnished reputations, and collapsed dynasties. Because of its pejorative connotations, the term was recast more positively a few years ago as *erectile dysfunction* (ED), which better defines the condition and has since been accepted internationally.

Approximately 152 million men worldwide—a figure projected to increase to over 320 million by the year 2025—needlessly suffer from the inability to achieve or maintain an erection sufficiently rigid for successful penetration and subsequent orgasm and ejaculation. It has been estimated that ED, to different degrees of severity, may affect more than 50% of the world's men over the age of 40 and may be particularly bothersome to a third of them.

Statistics show that approximately 12.5% of the male population in the United States, or about 20–30 million men—including up to about 52% of men 40 to 70 years old—currently suffer from sexual dysfunction. Statistics further reveal that almost all men will, at one time or another, experience temporary episodes of inability to perform sexually. Although the great majority of adults of all ages view sexual activity as a key issue for optimal quality of life, sexual dysfunction is underreported, misdiagnosed, and poorly treated in the

United States and all over the world—despite being a major cause of marital discord and, probably, divorce.

The sexually dysfunctional man finds his life shattered by his problem. He loses confidence and self-esteem. He is anxious, stressed, depressed, and may feel inadequate. His sense of manhood, his virility, and his self-image are bruised. Tension develops between the man and his partner and may emerge in his professional performance as well. Disharmony appears in his relationships with family and friends. He may deny the problem or shift the blame to his partner. Often, ED leads to total avoidance of any sexual activity or relationship, resulting in complete abstinence for fear of failure and embarrassment.

With the revolutionary discovery of the phosphodiesterase type 5 inhibitors, such as Viagra (sildenafil), Cialis (tadalafil), and Levitra (vardenafil), and the use of these oral medications by millions of men with excellent results and only a few minor side effects, a new era has dawned for the successful and safe management of ED. This recent advance has markedly increased people's awareness of sexual disorders, and it has helped a large number of men and women to discuss the issue socially and in the mass media without any shame or embarrassment. It has also encouraged millions of men in all parts of the world to seek the new drug therapies, resulting in a very high satisfaction rate and marked improvement in the psychological and emotional disturbances associated with ED.

Ironically, treatment success has also caused some marital problems, due to the sudden resurrection of potency in men who, after ignoring sex for a long time, have recovered their sexual prowess. Their sexual rejuvenation may not be welcomed by wives who are postmenopausal and/or may have lost interest in sex. Conflict may arise between husbands who feel sexually born again and wives who are unhappy or indifferent at the prospect of sexual activity—particularly when, after years of abstinence, men feel proud to be able to offer their partners an opportunity to revive the flame of desire and passion from the ashes of inadequacy and dysfunction, only to be met with apprehension, dislike, and rejection. This sadly common phenomenon may contribute to many cases of adultery and divorce and has doubtless strained the foundation of many formerly solid marriages.

Furthermore, some men suffer from what has been termed "Viagravation," stemming originally from low sexual desire and a lack of interest in sex, which is then confounded by the new and simple means of regaining normal sexual functioning with the help of a pill. These men experience a lot of pressure to resume sexual activity, which they subconsciously reject and for which they do not nurture any interest. Although they may at times comply with their partners' demands for sex, it will be without much conviction or desire. They may fail in their attempts because of deep anxiety and a lack of the sexual stimulation that is essential for the success of this particular pharmacologic therapy.

The medical community's understanding of sexual dysfunction's physiology, pathophysiology, and etiology continues to evolve. Since my 1994 publication of *Perfect Lover*, first edition, newer, safer, more effective methods for the diagnosis and treatment of ED have been established. These methods offer excellent opportunities for the sexually dysfunctional man to overcome his problem and resume a fulfilling, satisfying, healthy sex life at almost any age, and even despite his affliction by several chronic diseases (as long as his general medical condition allows for sexual activity without any risks). Unfortunately, however, fewer than 12% of the men who presently suffer from persistent inability to achieve and/or maintain an erection sufficient for satisfactory sexual activity are receiving any medical treatment for it. Instead, they accept or ignore the agony of their condition out of fear, ignorance, shame, embarrassment, selfishness, and various cultural or ethnic beliefs.

Today's men with sexual dysfunction have the opportunity to acquire an understanding of all effective modern therapies for their condition. A basic sex education is important for their partners as well. Not only may they harbor their own sexual problems, but they have a vested interest in their partners' restoration to good working order—especially because, as demonstrated in a recent study, sexual disturbance is a major cause of marital problems in the Western world.

Proper education and a high level of public awareness are crucial to dispelling myths and misperceptions concerning normal sexual function and its disturbances. I hope to provide answers to your current questions, and also to instill a desire to raise more questions. It is by asking and seeking that the reader may best benefit from this book.

The information in this book encompasses a thorough review of the literature, scientific presentations at American and international meetings, and my personal experience of more than 35 years treating thousands of patients suffering from this psychologically devastating medical condition. My intent is to present the most comprehensive, up-to-date, single-reference source possible on the subject of male sexual dysfunction and to provide my readers, be they medical professionals or laypersons, with better insight into this problem.

I have also attempted to make the material on a complex subject as simple and readable as possible and to ensure that the language herein reflects my awareness that interpersonal relationships other than between a husband and wife are affected by male sexual dysfunction. I hope I have succeeded.

Chapter One

SEXUAL EVOLUTION AND REVOLUTION

Sex is the gateway to life.

R. Harris

Among the many historical and cultural figures known to have been afflicted with sexual disorders are Richard I, Louis XVI, Napoleon I, Don Carlos II, George Bernard Shaw, Ludwig van Beethoven, and Johannes Brahms. Other prominent people, both reputable and shady, have more recently turned public attention to male sexual dysfunction. Senator Bob Dole admitted his sexual difficulty following a radical prostatectomy for prostate cancer and attributed its successful management to the use of Viagra. "Godfather" Paul Castellano's erectile dysfunction (ED) and its treatment with a penile prosthesis was documented in a book by two former Federal Bureau of Investigation agents.

Humanity's understanding of sex and its dysfunctions has markedly improved over the last 10 years, thanks to great strides in clarifying sexual physiology, pathophysiology, and pathogenesis. Historical interest in the subject can be traced back for thousands of years, but for a proper perspective on recent revolutionary developments, it is helpful to look even further back, into millions of years of sexual evolution.

FROM ANIMAL TO MAN: ERECTILE AND SEXUAL EVOLUTION

At one time, our human ancestors may have had a bone in the penis, which gave it permanent rigidity and a state of continuous erection. Over time, and for practical reasons, the bone, or os penis, disappeared as men began to walk erect. As man's penis became a flaccid organ, its sexual control was turned over to a higher center, the brain, a development that differentiates him from most other animals. The brain can facilitate or inhibit the human erectile process. Any time the brain releases its inhibitive control, spontaneous erections can occur.

Many animals still retain the os penis. In the whale, the bone measures about 6 feet in length and about 15 inches in circumference. In other mammals, such as the dog, fox, or bear, its size is less than 1 inch. The lion has a retractable penis, giving it good protection from injury. Snakes, on the other hand, have two penises, which they use interchangeably. One can also serve as a spare if something happens to the other.

Contrary to much male fantasizing, there is no practical advantage (for humans, anyway) in having two penises if one is functioning and can carry out that function satisfactorily. Some male animals, in fact, engage in sexual activity quite successfully without a penis. The male sea horse has a pouch, while the female has a penis. During intercourse, the female penetrates and releases her ova into this pouch, which is full of the male's sperms; the male thus becomes pregnant. Many male birds also have pouches and are without penises.

The modern human penis is mainly composed of fibroelastic erectile tissue, which has three principle parts. Two of these, a side-by-side set of spongy tissue chambers called the corpora cavernosa, comprise the largest portion of penile space and are the major erectile components of the penis. The third and smaller spongy part is the corpus spongiosum, which occupies the underside of the penis and covers the urethra (urinary channel). Those spongy parts, which form a frame for the vascular spaces and vessels, are surrounded by muscles and a firm sheath (Figure 1.1). At the external distal end of these is the cone-shaped glans penis, or head.

Despite containing no bone and occurring singly, the human penis, in shape and anatomy, is far superior to those of other animals. It can easily penetrate and ejaculate directly into the female vagina; it is well protected from trauma; and on erection, it attains a size relatively larger than that of most other animals. It not only serves to pass urine and semen but also becomes erect, thereby allowing the man to engage in sexual activity when the opportunity arises. Beyond those bodily functions, it leads a rather sedate and idle life. But it is fascinating to observe the obsession most human males have with their penises—its size, length, and girth, and its erectile capabilities. This preoccupation, as it turns out, is nothing new.

The Penis in Ancient Art and Philosophy

The penis has been drawn, painted, and sculpted for millions of years by hundreds of civilizations. Many ancient cultures were most appreciative of

Figure 1.1
Anatomy of the Human Penis

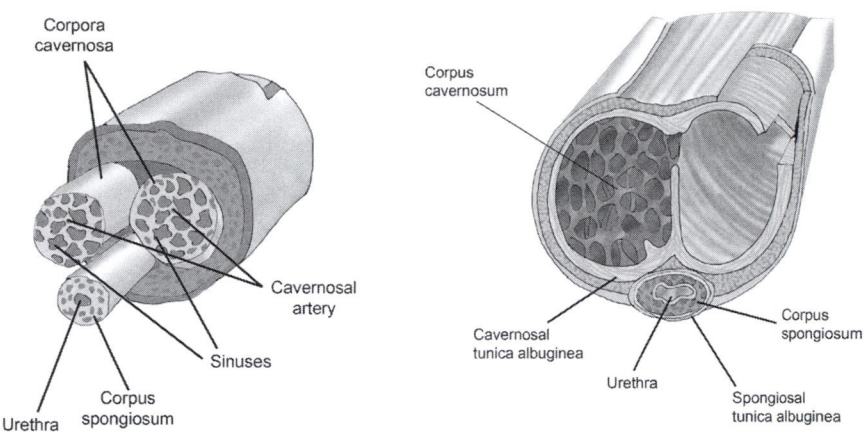

Courtesy of Alexander Balmaceda.

the large penis. Early Hindu culture exhibits this admiration in its well-hung male sculptures and other artwork. Interestingly, however, this worship did not extend to living humans, in whom the smaller penis was favored. The famous Hindu *Kama Sutra*, written by an Indian scholar between 330 and 369 A.D., is well known as a sex manual describing various postures and positions for lovemaking as well as psychological aspects of the interactions and scenarios of love (Lue TF et al. 2004b)—but the *Kama Sutra* also defines categories of men by their penile size. The man with a 2- to 3-inch erect penis ("rabbit man") is depicted as lithe and strong, the ideal lover. The man with a 4- to 6-inch erect penis ("deer man") is fleet and graceful, the perfect warrior. The least admired is the rare male with a thick, bulky, 9-inch or longer erect penis ("stallion man"), who is considered worthless and indolent.

In Pharaonic Egypt, the erect penis depicted in many murals and statues was a symbol of strength and good fortune. Greek gods were portrayed with enormous endowments as well, although common human males were portrayed with significantly smaller organs, as the early Greeks considered large penises in mere mortals to be abnormal and ungainly. The philosopher Aristotle (384–322 B.C.) also held that a man with a shorter penis was more fertile, reasoning that semen traveling a shorter distance did not have a chance to "cool off."

In many cultures the erect penis was considered as the "symbol of masculinity, strength, endurance, courage, ability, intelligence, knowledge, symbol of loving and being loved, possession of women and dominance over men" (Wylie KR, Eardley I 2007). Various primitive methods were used to lengthen and widen the penis. The Topinama of Brazil used snakebites on their penises to enlarge them for a few months, while the Indian Sadhus tried to lengthen them with weights. The Dayak tribesmen pierced the glans penis and introduced objects into the holes to achieve maximal stimulation of their partners (Talalaj J, Talalaj S 1994).

Erectile Dysfunction (ED) and Its Empirical Management through the Centuries

Male sexual dysfunction is as old as the world. The Bible attributed it to a divine curse. The Greek physician and so-called father of medicine, Hippocrates (460–375 B.C.), attributed ED to man's professional preoccupations and the ugliness of the female. Eighteenth- and nineteenth-century religious moralists maintained that it was caused by excessive sexual activities such as masturbation, prostitution, and promiscuity. ED has been "treated" over the years by witchcraft, exorcism, and religious counseling. Fortunately, ignorance and superstition about sexual function and dysfunction were eventually superceded (at least to some extent) by scientific examination and discovery.

The mechanism of erection was first described by the famous Italian artist and inventor Leonardo da Vinci (1452–1519)—himself a sufferer of ED— who related it to the filling of the penis with blood. The physician Costanzo Varolio (1543–1575) later described the erectile function of the muscles surrounding the penis, although the very first description of these muscles is attributed to the Greek physician Galen in the second century A.D.

Chinese, Greek, Roman, and Egyptian literatures mention numerous potions to increase sexual potency. Historical remedies for ED have included the ingestion of animal testes and testicular extracts—and this is not as far off the mark as it may sound. In 1889, French physiologist Charles Edouard Brown-Sequard injected himself with extracts made of blood from the testicular vein, semen, and a liquid obtained from crushing the testicles of young dogs and guinea pigs. He reported an excellent sexual response to this cocktail, considered by many experts to be the birth of male hormone therapy.

LILLY-ICOS AND THE HISTORY OF HUMAN SEXUALITY

Since ancient times, men and women have been aware of their lust and basic urge to fornicate. Sexual attitudes and activities have been defined and redefined for thousands of years by countless personal, religious, ethical, societal, and ethnic influences. At a recent annual meeting of the American Urological Association, Lilly-ICOS (the manufacturer of Cialis) distributed an elegant booklet titled *Sexuality: Perception and Performance throughout History,* illustrating the changing image and practice of sex over time and in various cultures (Patel 2006). Following are several interesting nuggets adapted from that booklet:

Ancient Humanity

Sex was simply a natural and enjoyable act of sensual pleasure, not influenced by moral or procreational considerations, until about 9000 B.C. With the male role in reproduction unknown, the woman was the epicenter of the family. Men's reproductive contribution was acknowledged around the time that people moved into villages with supplies of vegetation and livestock. Producing numerous offspring for more field hands was highly desirable in those agricultural societies, so a woman's inability to conceive was a blemish that cast her in a subordinate role.

Early Egypt

Marriage with girls as young as 12 was common. Contraception was practiced with lotions and other concoctions, interruption of coitus before ejaculation, anal sex, sex with animals, and the insertion of substances such as honey and crocodile dung into the vagina to prevent sperms' passage to the cervix.

Early Greece

Men often satisfied sexual urges by means of homosexual behavior and pederasty, especially with young postpubertal boys. Women often sought gratification through masturbation or lesbian sex. Women were considered inferior to men and classified into three groups: wives for procreation, concubines for sexual gratification, and high-class prostitutes for sexual and intellectual stimulation.

Roman Empire

Sexual liberalism, prostitution, public baths for men and women, and mythological sexual deities reflected the Romans' "insouciant and nonchalant attitude toward sex" and widespread promiscuity, which persisted until the fall of the Empire. With the eventual domination of the Christian church, sex for pleasure (rather than procreation), homosexuality, masturbation, and contraception were condemned as sinful and were banned, sometimes by violent means.

Early India

The teachings of the aforementioned *Kama Sutra* (aphorisms of pleasure) focused on *artha,* or material well-being, and *kama,* or pleasure and love. Sex was considered a religious duty to be treated with respect and great consideration, an art to be acquired through practice, and an emotional act of love's expression. Along with instructions for both men and women in various sexual techniques for maximal pleasure, the manual provided lists of aphrodisiacs and modes of contraception. Indian culture's high regard for marriage was reflected in the custom of *sati,* in which a widow committed suicide by throwing herself on her husband's funeral pyre to accompany him in death.

Early Islamic World

Women who were classified as respectable ladies were admired and sheltered in harems to protect them from the so-called evils of society. These harems also provided men with the opportunity to have sex at will with numerous women. Fifteenth-century Turks built the Grand Turk, a small city for the 300–1,200 concubines in the sultan's harem, which gave him a vast choice of partners to choose from for his sexual gratification. A fifteenth- or sixteenth-century sex manual titled *The Perfumed Garden for the Soul's Recreation* detailed explicit methods for successful intercourse and remedies for sexual problems.

Early China

The Taoist doctrine emphasized the importance of sex for enjoying a long, healthy life and as means for the couple to complement each other and connect spiritually. Women represented the source of an inexhaustible yin essence, which men, with their easily depleted yang essence, needed to absorb to achieve harmony and prolong their lives. The man was encouraged to engage in as much sex with as many partners as possible to stockpile yin, while also conserving yang through various methods of preventing ejaculation. Several manuals on sexual techniques, positions, and foreplay were available, as well as tonics and lotions to increase sexual pleasure and methods to elongate the penis and shrink the vagina. Masturbation and homosexuality were forbidden for men but allowed for women. Later, the philosopher Confucius attacked sexual promiscuity and imposed moral views that sanctioned marriage but allowed men to have multiple wives to produce sons. Although Confucius expressed disdain for women, he insisted on the man's obligation to fulfill the sexual desires of his wives and concubines. Confucianism's rigid regulations persisted until the mid-seventeenth century.

Renaissance Europe

Despite the church's prohibitions, rigid constraints, and condemnation of premarital sex (which was widespread nevertheless), this age, particularly in Italy, was marked by sexual liberalism and the dominance of sexuality in art, with nudity depicted in paintings, sculptures, and murals. A large number of illegitimate children and a high incidence of sexually transmitted diseases (STDs) were recorded, leading to the development and use of the condom.

Sixteenth- to Nineteenth-Century Japan

The "pleasure quarters" flourished with regulated prostitution, several published manuals called *shunga* gave specific instructions on lovemaking techniques (especially for newlyweds), and the famed Japanese geishas provided customers with incomparable entertainment in music, song, and dance.

Nineteenth-Century Europe and America

Sexual liberalism and promiscuity were widespread, nudity was again prominent in art, and prostitution was prevalent all over Europe and the United States in the 1800s. A steep increase in STDs reached about 30,000 cases in London in 1850s. This trend persisted to the next century, with gonorrhea affecting half the male population in the United States by 1914 and reaching about 100 million cases by 1970, prompting the British and U.S. governments to form antiprostitution statutes.

The Twentieth Century

Feminism and women's liberation movements contributed to a liberal attitude toward sex unrestricted by moral or religious prohibitions. This attitude promoted the development of different forms of contraception, which allowed for sexual freedom, but was accompanied by a markedly increased incidence of STDs, including AIDS.

And so the worldwide evolution and revolution of human sexuality continues…

Man's Penile Obsession

In a healthy state, the human penis is a very efficient tool for maximum sexual gratification, procreation, and perpetuation of the species. But even when the penis is capable of doing what it is designed to do, and does it effectively, men may have any number of complaints: that it's too short, too narrow, ugly, that it curves the wrong way—even that it's too big or too long. In other words, those men want it to be something it is not.

Aside from the exceptions afforded by modern medical and surgical techniques, what a man is born with is what he must live with for the rest of his life. Because of their previously mentioned fascination with penile characteristics and function, however, many men try to find ways to lengthen the penis. For some, their worry and embarrassment over penile size is so great that they become sexually dysfunctional. When the object of his pride then fails to respond, it is an uncompromising witness to a man's sexual failure. A man can fake sensitivity, caring, faithfulness, and many other human emotions—but one thing he cannot fake is an erection.

Micropenis: Myth or Reality?

Although the size of the penis varies from man to man, it probably has less relationship, physically or structurally, to other parts of a man's body than any other bodily component. Measurement of flaccid size may not be a valid test to assess the true length of the penis. Many men with large flaccid penises experience relatively little growth in erectness, whereas the man with a smaller flaccid penis sees a dramatic change in size on becoming erect.

Medically speaking, most so-called micropenises are actually normal sized and may simply be buried in the dense suprapubic fat (fatty tissue above the pubic bone) usually found in obese men. The procedure to lengthen these penises is relatively simple. When the suprapubic fat pad is pulled upward, the penis is usually found to have a normal length. For those men, exercise and diet alone may reduce the fat pad and provide natural penile elongation without the need for any medical or surgical treatment.

In exceptional cases, when the penis is truly small—measuring less than 1.8 inches in the flaccid state and less than 2.8 inches during erection—and especially if this is actually causing severe psychological disturbance, surgical elongation of the penis may be attempted in an effort to add about 1–2 inches to its length.

Unfortunately, several surgical techniques for lengthening and widening a short and narrow penis have proven largely unsuccessful, for example, dividing the suspensory ligaments that attach the base of the penis to the pubic bone; performing a V-Y plasty (making a V-shaped incision on the lower abdomen above the penile base, then closing the incision in a Y-shape); or taking fat from the lower abdomen and injecting it around the shaft of the penis. These techniques may commonly result in the development of inflammatory and scar tissue around the shaft, and even marked penile deformities, necessitating additional corrective surgery. (They have also led to well-publicized lawsuits, which have cost one particular urologist in California his medical license and millions of dollars in litigation.) However, as discussed in chapter 3, certain surgical procedures for penile enlargement, performed by experts, may lead to satisfactory results.

MEDICAL MILESTONES IN THE MANAGEMENT OF ED

Although history is replete with various exotic (and not so exotic) remedies for sexual dysfunction, effective treatment for ED was hindered for centuries by societal constraints, misconceptions, myths, and taboos. Rigid religious and political prohibitions against sexual expression and research persisted until the early 1900s, when psychologist Sigmund Freud of Vienna began to change attitudes toward sex by asserting that humans are sexual animals with the impulse to reproduce. In 1912, Freud made a major contribution with his book *The Most Prevalent Form of Degradation in Erotic Life*, discussing various psychological causes of sexual disorders. From that time forward, psychological and medical advances in the field of sexual dysfunction proceeded together.

The 1930s witnessed the identification and isolation of testosterone as the male sex hormone, and it was used rather indiscriminately to treat ED in the period 1935–1940. In 1948, Dr. Alfred Kinsey from Indiana published the results of his extensive, pioneering studies on human sexuality, *Sexual Behavior in the Human Male,* to great worldwide interest. This work and his subsequent books, by elucidating normal and abnormal sexual behavior in both men and women, improved the understanding of psychosocial and other factors controlling human sexual tendencies and expression.

In 1970, in their milestone book *Human Sexual Inadequacy,* doctors William Masters and Virginia Johnson highlighted the importance of performance anxiety as a primary cause of ED. They revolutionized the understanding of normal and abnormal sexual functioning and laid the foundation of sex therapy, stressing the necessity of treating the marital unit rather than the man alone. And in the early 1970s, the medical community began to accept penile prostheses for ED treatment.

Timeline: Vascular Surgery, Devices, Implants, and Injections

By the beginning of the twentieth century, urologists were showing interest in the penile vascular system and erectile failure, paying particular attention to issues of blood flow into the penis as well as premature or excessive outflow. The following timeline traces these developments.

1902   Wooten described improved erections from tying off the deep penile dorsal vein; Lydeton reported similar results in 1908.

1923   Leriche established that some ED was associated with vascular disease.

1973   Michal reported a new microvascular surgical technique for ED, consisting of anastomosis (joining) of the epigastric artery (located behind the lower abdominal rectus muscle) directly to the corpus cavernosa.

1982   Virag reported correcting penile arterial insufficiency by connecting the epigastric artery directly to the deep penile dorsal vein; this procedure was also found to correct overly rapid venous outflow.

1985   Wespes and Schulman reported erectile improvement from stripping and tying off the deep penile dorsal vein and its associated tributaries.

Subsequently, in an explosion of research that continued into the 1990s, several bypass procedures between the epigastric artery and the penile dorsal artery or vein were utilized to increase blood flow to the penis; for example, Furlow modified Virag's technique by tying off the distal penile vein. Experimental surgical procedures were also developed to locate and repair offending leaky veins, but despite relatively high short-term success, long-term results were disappointing. Nowadays, the leakage-related procedures are rarely performed, except in select cases of significant venous leakage between the corpus spongiosum and corpora cavernosa.

In the early twentieth century, Dr. Otto Lederer of Vienna patented a device to produce an erection with a vacuum. It did not, however, appear in established, peer-reviewed medical journals or win acceptance from the medical community. In the early 1960s, to treat his own ED, David Osbon Sr. of Georgia developed an externally applied vacuum device—apparently without knowledge of the previous Austrian invention—called the "Youth Equivalent Device," but made no attempt to market it until about 15 years later.

Meanwhile, penile prostheses progressed significantly, as follows.

1936   Bogaras used a section of rib cartilage to replace an amputated penis.

1948   Bergman used a rib graft to replace an amputated penis; however, it was found that such natural materials were eventually absorbed by the body, soon rendering the prosthesis nonfunctional.

1948   Bohayris produced a rigid plastic tube as an artificial os penis.

1952   Goodwin and Scott described a semirigid acrylic penile prosthesis.

1960   Behairi placed polyethylene implants into the corpora cavernosa; Loeffler placed acrylic implants into the penis outside the corpora.

1968   Lash placed a single silicone implant under the corpora cavernosa.

1972   Pearman used a single silastic prosthesis; he also implanted paired silicon rods; Subriñi used paired silicone rods the following year.

1973   In response to the demand for a more cosmetically appealing prosthesis, Scott and colleagues introduced an inflatable prosthesis.

1975   Small and colleagues used a pair of gel-filled silicone prostheses.

1977   Finney devised a hinged silicone prosthesis.

1980   Jonas introduced a silicone prosthesis containing embedded silver wires that allowed voluntary bending.

mid-1980s American Medical Systems (AMS) brought out a malleable, semirigid silicone rod with a stainless steel core; Dacomed brought out the Omniphase, a semirigid polyurethane prosthesis with a mechanically activated interlocking hinge; many new generations of inflatable prostheses have since been marketed by Surgitek, Mentor, Dacomed, and AMS.

Although the use of various agents to dilate blood vessels was already well known in medicine, the ability to induce erection by direct penile injection was stumbled on accidentally in 1972. Michal, while doing a revascularization of a patient's penile arteries, injected the vasodilator papaverine into the corpora cavernosa to increase the size of the blood vessels; to his surprise, an erection ensued. This finding led to further investigation and use of injectable vasodilators, as follows.

early 1980s   Virag and Brindley's independent studies suggested that intrapenile injections of certain vasodilators could be used in the treatment of ED.

1986   Intracavernous self-injection of vasoactive drugs became the predominant therapy for ED.

late 1980s   Prostaglandin E1 (PGE1) appeared on the scene.

early 1990s   A mixture of papaverine, phentolamine, PGE1, and, occasionally, forskolin was introduced; it appeared to produce better, more prolonged erections, with possibly fewer side effects.

Outcome studies of intrapenile injection, however, then revealed a high dropout rate due to men's apprehension toward injecting vasodilators directly into the penis. So, in 1998, a tiny intraurethral PGE1 insert was introduced. Unfortunately, its preliminary high success rate of about 65% declined to about 35% when the insert was used clinically on a large scale.

So-called Miracle Drugs

Oral medications, such as trazodone, arginine, delequamine, naltrexone, and nalmefene, were tried in the management of ED, but without success. Despite the other therapeutic options available, men with ED eagerly awaited the discovery of an ideal, noninvasive treatment with the following characteristics: "It should be simple to use and preferably by mouth, highly effective in all attempts of sexual intercourse, non-painful, with minimal side effects and at a low cost" (Hanash KA 1997).

Then, in 1998, a medical volcano erupted worldwide with Pfizer's introduction of a new drug called Viagra (sildenafil) for the management of ED. This compound, from the family of phosphodiesterase type 5 (PDE-5) inhibitors, was initially tested in the United Kingdom in 1992 for its coronary vasodilatory effects, particularly for the treatment of coronary artery disease and hypertension. To the surprised delight of the researchers (and Pfizer), several patients involved in the study reported improved sexual potency. This fortunate development—one of the great medical achievements of the century—shifted Viagra researchers' focus from the heart to the penis. Subsequent international studies reported excellent results with its use for ED management, with minor side effects.

An evolving understanding of brain biochemistry and the importance of the neurotransmitter dopamine in the erectile process led to the development and marketing of apomorphine in 2001. This drug resembles dopamine biochemically and acts directly on the brain's sexual centers to elicit an erection. Apomorphine achieved encouraging preliminary results with very few side effects but did not live up to expectations. Subsequent studies demonstrated poor efficacy, with a declining success rate of only 35% to 47%, compared to 32% for placebo.

In 2003, two new competitors in the family of PDE-5 inhibitors, Levitra (vardenafil) from Bayer-Glaxo, and Cialis (tadalafil) from Lilly-ICOS, stormed the market after approval by the U.S. Food and Drug Administration. Although the three drugs are chemically similar, Viagra, Levitra, and Cialis differ in their speed and duration of action, and in some of their side effects. Despite the high success rates obtained with all of these PDE-5 inhibitors, studies show a high dropout rate after a few months of using them. It seems that the majority of ED patients and their partners still want a treatment to restore their sexual functioning in a more natural way, without needing to rely on an artificial means (like medication) every time they plan to have sex.

Innovations on the Horizon

In some German studies, the daily use of PDE-5 inhibitors for several months has been found to restore sexual potency without the need for further treatment in over 55% of patients. Combined administration of PDE-5 inhibitors with intracorporeal injection of vasodilators or intraurethral insertion of PGE1 has also yielded good results. Furthermore, some men (particularly diabetics) for whom PDE-5 inhibitors previously failed have responded well to PDE-5 inhibitors taken along with hormone replacement therapy for decreased serum testosterone. Conversely, some men with ED and low testosterone who did not initially respond to hormone therapy have been able to develop good erections once PDE-5 inhibitors were added to their treatment.

As we enter the twenty-first century, many of the ED treatments currently in use have not yet been appraised in terms of their long-term effectiveness or unforeseen complications. Several new medications in the form of tablets, nasal sprays, and penile ointments are under study and will soon be available. One of the most promising new treatment modalities is gene therapy, transferring the genes for the production of pro-erectile substances, such as nitric oxide synthase or caveolin, directly into the corpora cavernosa. In animals and in selected men with ED, the preliminary results of gene therapy are encouraging, restoring normal erections for months, or even permanently. Another promising method is the use of adipose tissue–derived stem cells, which showed great potential in differentiating into urothelium, smooth muscle, blood vessel, and striated muscle when injected into the corpora of rats with type 2 diabetes mellitus and neurogenic ED. They significantly improved erectile function in these animals (Lue TF 2007).

The final chapters in the history of male sexual dysfunction and its treatment have not yet been written. As the issue receives more publicity, more men are willing to come forward and seek assistance, and medical science must contend with a steady supply of sexual problems for which permanent solutions remain to be discovered. In particular, significant research into the structure and physiology of penile smooth muscle, and preventive measures that would either delay or prevent the occurrence of ED, remain virgin territory.

ECSTASY AND AGONY

It is normal for every individual to be interested in and search for love and sex. Civilized man has molded his cultural temperament and lifestyle on ever-expanding concepts of love, sex, and passion, endlessly cultivating these concepts to thrive and grow. But despite increasing sophistication, mankind continuously encounters physical, psychological, and social difficulties in the expression of sexual desire and aspirations. Problems related to sex have multiplied, and tragedies of failure occur in increasingly significant numbers.

Modern man—and woman—should be better prepared for the art of sex and love. Men and women deserve to regard and experience sex as a pleasurable act with an overt emotional display. It also has many physical and mental health benefits. The following chapters explore various aspects of sex and its dysfunctions and provide a global, up-to-date review of the causes and effects of these disorders and current methods for their diagnosis and treatment.

Chapter Two

SEX EDUCATION

Sex is the foundation of marriage. Yet most married couples do not know the ABC of sex.

T. H. Van der Weld

No book on sexual problems could be considered complete if it did not address sex education. This important subject has great impact not only on the future sexual behavior of teenagers, but also on understanding the etiologies of sexual disturbances in adults. Yet in many cultures, the subject is taboo, prohibited from discussion or even mentioning in conversation. It is quite frustrating to realize that ignorance of the fundamentals of sex prevails among adolescents and adults worldwide.

Adolescents generally acquire most of their sex education from peers, magazines, television, and movies, and in some parts of the Western world, at school. In general, parents are reluctant to discuss sexual matters with their children out of embarrassment, ignorance, discomfort, or fear of encouraging sexual activity—and if they do talk about sex, they often resort to well-established euphemisms. Jewel Akens wrote the song "The Birds and the Bees" to address youngsters about sex and love, emphasizing, "It's time you learned about the facts of life starting from A to Z." Clichés aside, we should heed his advice. Parents must be encouraged to assume this responsibility, demonstrating an open willingness to guide their teenagers on a path of proper adaptation to their emerging sexuality.

It behooves all parents to be actively involved in their children's sexual maturation by showing trust and providing good advice. They should complement all the information provided at school and clarify for their teenagers the meaning and values of sex (Schaalma HP et al. 2004). If they are unable to answer some of the questions raised—which is to be expected, and is only natural—they should not be embarrassed to admit it, and to look up the answers in specialized books or consult their family physicians.

This chapter provides concise and clear information about some of the most common issues pertaining to sex education, not only for adolescents, but also for adults who may find themselves lacking sufficient knowledge in this area. It is not my intention to present a comprehensive review, but rather to offer some guidelines for parents who are trying to answer their children's questions about sex, and to help them illuminate their youngsters' minds about clean, healthy, joyful sexuality.

WHY IS SEX EDUCATION SO IMPORTANT?

The major goals of sex education are to do the following:

• Provide a framework for safe and clean sexual health
• Encourage the development of sound, acceptable social and sexual skills
• Teach about the anatomy and physiology of male and female genitalia
• Discuss the risks and consequences of consensual and nonvolitional sex
• Provide accurate information about the dangers of unprotected sexual activity
• Stress the importance of safe sex practices

Sex education also aims to present a true image of sex and to dispel all the misperceptions, taboos, and myths related to it, as these may play a major role in producing certain sexual disturbances later in life.

WHO SHOULD BE RESPONSIBLE FOR THE SEX EDUCATION OF CHILDREN AND ADOLESCENTS?

In the United States and several other Western countries, sex education is part of many schools' curricula. Despite their best efforts, however, these courses or programs may not address all aspects of sexuality; for example, they may lack the expertise or scope to cover the social skills relevant to healthy sexual and romantic relationships. Sex educators should emphasize that students' parents have a crucial responsibility and role in establishing solid rules and principles regarding future sexual activity and all of its potential risks.

AT WHAT AGE SHOULD CHILDREN BE PROVIDED WITH SEX EDUCATION BY THEIR PARENTS?

It is never too early for parents to start talking with their children about sexual behavior and answering their questions about it in an open, honest, and comfortable way, tailored to the child's level of maturity and understanding. For preschoolers and school-aged children, the information is best provided not as a lengthy and boring lecture, but in recurring smaller conversations. Parents should not overwhelm their youngsters with too much information at one time, but rather spread it over many months—golden opportunities to broach the subject will inevitably arise.

HOW SHOULD PARENTS ANSWER THEIR CHILDREN'S QUESTIONS ABOUT SEXUAL TOPICS?

Answers should be accurate, short, and candid, providing precise and simple information in exact terms (penis, vagina, uterus, and such) to explain sex organs, sexual behaviors and functions, and pregnancy. Parents should welcome all inquiries, even when they do not know all the answers or feel uncomfortable. They should appoint themselves as the ultimate resource for all sexual matters and promise to research the correct answers and information. This will show children and teenagers that sex is an acceptable topic of discussion and that their parents can be relied on for honest answers to sexual questions.

IF CHILDREN DO NOT SHOW ANY INTEREST IN SEX EDUCATION, HOW CAN PARENTS BRING IT UP WITHOUT ALIENATING THEM?

It is not always easy to get a child to discuss sexual issues. Parents may need a lot of tact, patience, and perseverance to break this particular ice. If a child or teenager seems unwilling to listen to any information or engage in instructional conversation on the subject, a parent may have to seize any opportunity—after a movie, during a long car ride, sharing a snack—to broach the topic more informally, perhaps by asking about his or her friends' opinions regarding a sexual matter. Parents who feel at all uncomfortable about this should prepare themselves for any potential awkwardness by rehearsing beforehand.

"WHERE DO BABIES COME FROM?"

A question commonly asked by children of all ages, this can be embarrassing for parents to address but should elicit honest answers tailored to the child's level of maturity and ability to understand. As children get older, the clichés involving birds, bees, and storks should be gradually replaced by simple, accurate, and straightforward information. Here is an example of an answer—which may be one of thousands—that could satisfy a youngster's curiosity:

> You know how much Mom and Dad, like so many married couples, love each other? To bless our union and our deep affection, God gave us the power to bring a new

person into the world who will be the fruit of our love. So Mom was created with ovaries where eggs are formed, and Dad with testicles that can produce sperms, which look like tiny fish with a tail. Dad's sperms can penetrate Mom's eggs and start creating a baby, who will grow in Mom's womb until it's time to be born.

It may not even be necessary to go into further details about how the sperms met the eggs through sexual intercourse, depending on the extent of the child's curiosity. However, parents should be ready to furnish additional information on that subject if requested, and to do so comfortably and without apparent embarrassment.

IS SEX DIRTY?

Sex, properly used and not abused, is beautiful. It is God's gift to all humans to experience this ultimate sensual pleasure. How boring life would be without sex! Consensual sex is like fresh snow, a morning breeze, a rainbow, a full moon, or a melodious symphony. It is the foundation of marriage and perpetuates the human race. As beautifully stated by Dr. Havelock Ellis, "Sexual pleasure, wisely used and not abused, may prove the stimulus and liberation of our finest and most exalted activities" (Havelock E 1922, 118).

However, sex can become dirty, filthy, and criminal when it is forced on someone. Sex should not be accepted out of fear, obligation, threat, or revenge. Rape or other sexual abuse of children is a hideous crime. A common aspect of forced sex nowadays is date rape; this often involves the impairment of judgment by alcohol or drugs and can have serious physical and psychological consequences.

Every teenager should be warned about sexual abuse, date rape, pornography (including child pornography), drugs, and alcohol. Furthermore, it behooves parents to stress to their younger children that although it is acceptable for them to touch their own genitalia (see the following section), they should categorically refuse to be sexually touched, and they must refrain from sexually touching anybody else.

IS MASTURBATION HARMFUL?

There is no medical evidence that masturbation, as practiced by almost all children, adolescents, and adults (including married people), is medically harmful. It certainly does not cause the growth of hair on the palms or horns on the head! It does not cause dementia, convulsions, impotence, infertility, or any other physical or mental disease—provided, however, that it is not abused and does not ultimately become a person's only means of sexual gratification, completely replacing other forms of normal sexual activity. If masturbation is practiced excessively, such as several times a day, it may lead to an obsessive-compulsive behavior involving serious psychological and sexual disturbance (such as retarded or absent ejaculation or orgasm during sexual intercourse, but not during masturbation).

The bottom line: although it is perfectly normal for a child to explore his or her body, and to masturbate occasionally, whether for pleasure or for relief of boredom or stress, children must be instructed not to make it an excessive habit and that masturbating in public or on other children or adults is strictly prohibited.

WHAT IS A BRIEF, ACCURATE DESCRIPTION OF THE MALE GENITALIA?

The external male genitalia (see Figure 2.1) consist of the penis, which serves as a tool for erection, penetration, and ejaculation as well as for the passage of urine; the testicles, which serve as factories for sperms and the male hormone testosterone; and the scrotum, which harbors the testicles and works as a thermostat to keep testicular temperature about 4.5°F below body temperature.

The internal male genitalia include the Cowper's glands in the urethra, which secrete a fluid during sexual excitement responsible for washing out the urine from the urethra and for the lubrication of the glans penis for easier intromission into the vagina, and which may also contain some sperms; the prostate gland, which produces some of the seminal fluid that contains essential

Figure 2.1
Male External and Internal Genitalia

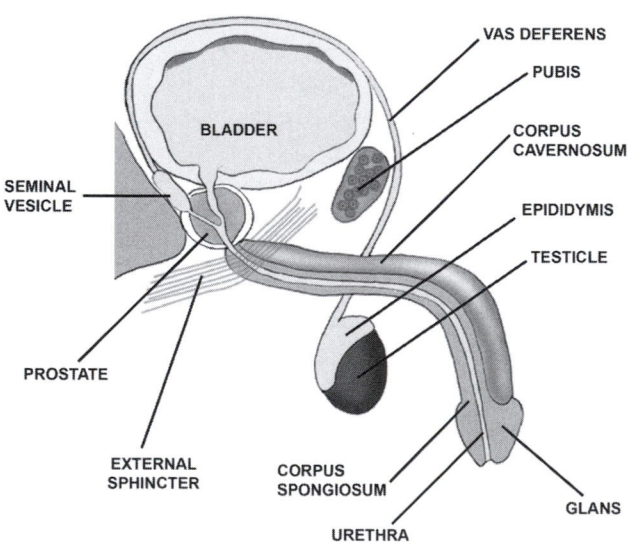

Courtesy of Alexander Balmaceda.

nutrients for sperms' survival and activity; the seminal vesicles (behind the prostate), which secrete the bulk of the seminal fluid; the epididymi (behind and alongside the testicles), which contain the maturing sperms; and the vasa deferentia, which are conduits for the ejection of sperms and semen through the penis during ejaculation. (See a following section for more on puberty.)

WHAT IS A BRIEF, ACCURATE DESCRIPTION OF THE FEMALE GENITALIA?

The external female genitalia include the labia majora (two elongated skin folds running from the lower part of the pubic bone to the lower end of the vaginal outlet); the labia minora (two smaller folds around the external vaginal opening, or vulva); the vagina (extending from the vulva to the internal uterine opening, or cervix), a canal that receives the penis during intercourse and serves in the monthly passage of menstrual blood and the delivery of the baby at the end of pregnancy; and the clitoris (above the opening of the urinary channel, the urethra), which is very sensitive to sexual stimulation.

Figure 2.2
Female Internal and External Genitalia

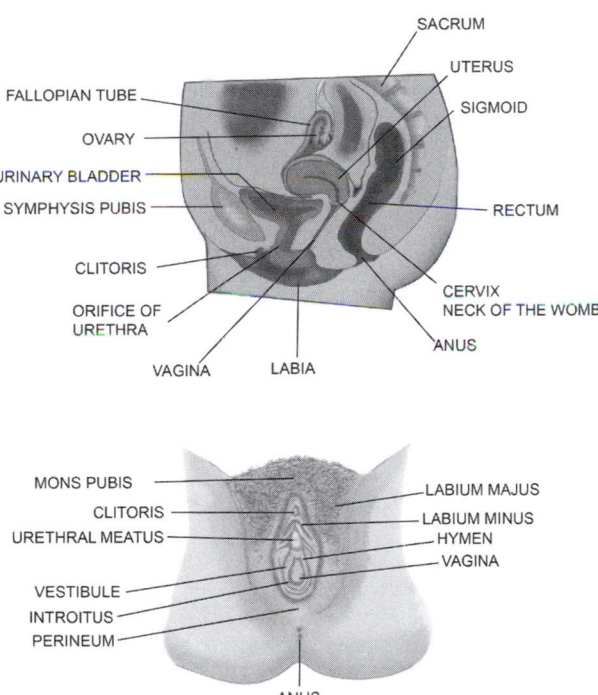

Courtesy of Alexander Balmaceda.

The female internal genitalia (see Figure 2.2) consist of the ovaries (alongside the uterus and against the bony pelvic wall), which secrete the female hormones, contain ovarian follicles that house ova (eggs) at various stages of their maturation, and release ova approximately monthly; the fallopian tubes (extending from the ovaries to the uterus), through which mature ova travel; and the uterus (a hollow, muscular organ connected to the cervix), which builds up a lining that develops into a placenta if pregnancy occurs or drains out in menstruation otherwise. (See a following section for more on puberty and menstruation.)

An ovum (egg) released from its follicle may encounter sperms in the fallopian tube or uterus if sexual intercourse has recently occurred. The cervix is the gate through which sperms can enter the uterus from the vagina; during pregnancy, it is normally closed to hold the fetus up, and it opens for delivery.

WHAT ARE THE PHYSICAL CHANGES THAT OCCUR IN BOYS AT PUBERTY?

Puberty is the period during which a surge in production of gender-specific (in this case, male) sex hormones causes the development of secondary sex characteristics and the ability to reproduce sexually. In human males, from about seven years old to adulthood, increased secretion of luteinizing hormone (LH) from the brain's pituitary gland stimulates production of testosterone by the testicles. Testosterone production peaks around 10–12 years of age. This causes boys to experience several physical changes, usually between the ages of 12 and 17: hoarseness and deepening of the voice; growth of pubic, facial, and body hair; enlargement of the penis and testicles; increased sexual desire; firm erections; and the ability to ejaculate semen containing millions of sperms that are capable of fertilizing a female's egg.

WHAT ARE THE PHYSICAL CHANGES THAT OCCUR IN GIRLS AT PUBERTY?

Puberty is the period during which a surge in production of gender-specific (in this case, female) sex hormones causes the development of secondary sex characteristics and the ability to reproduce sexually. Under the influence of hormones secreted by the brain's pituitary gland, the maturing ovaries begin secreting the female hormones, usually around 12–14 years of age. This causes girls to experience physical changes such as increased height, increased growth of pubic and body hair, breast development, and menstruation. Once menstruation occurs, a girl is physically mature enough to become pregnant (see the following section).

WHAT CAUSES MENSTRUATION, AND WHAT IS ITS PURPOSE?

Most girls start menstruating around 12–13 years of age, although they may begin as early as 9 or as late as 15. Monthly bleeding varies from one girl to another. Within an individual, it may vary from one cycle to the next in amount, duration, time of occurrence, and degree of pain and other symptoms (like bloating, fatigue, and irritability). The usual span of the human menstrual cycle is around 28 days.

Normally, each month (usually about 14 days prior to the upcoming menstrual cycle), one of the two ovaries releases a mature ovum into the adjoining fallopian tube, an event called ovulation. Meanwhile, for several days before ovulation, under the influence of peak levels of LH and follicular stimulating hormone, secreted by the pituitary gland, and estrogen from the ovaries, the lining of the uterus thickens in preparation for a possible pregnancy.

If the ovum is not fertilized by a sperm, the bloodstream's concentration of the pituitary and ovarian hormones falls, and the extra uterine lining sloughs off, breaking down into a mixture of blood and tissue debris (including the unfertilized egg), which passes out though the vagina as menstrual bleeding.

On the other hand, if the ovum is fertilized and embeds in the uterus, thereby initiating pregnancy, estrogen and progesterone maintain their high levels in the bloodstream, the uterine lining develops into a placenta to support and nourish the growing fetus, and the menstrual cycle ceases for the duration of the pregnancy.

Menstruating girls (and their mothers) need accurate medical information about these natural physiological phenomena. Many girls are apprehensive or afraid of the onset of monthly bleeding; they may be concerned about hygiene, the possibility of severe menstrual pain, and more. Most of the information they receive is provided at school or volunteered by their friends, and it is not always accurate.

It behooves a mother to prepare her daughter for this life event and to dispel her fears about it, even if the girl is embarrassed and reluctant to talk about it (as most are). Rather than lecturing, have small conversations about menstruation, and encourage your daughter to feel comfortable discussing it. The subject can be broached casually and tactfully by asking her what she already knows about it.

WHAT ABOUT TEENAGERS AND HOMOSEXUALITY OR BISEXUALITY?

Many teenagers wonder and worry about being homosexual or bisexual, especially if they have crushes on individuals of the same sex or if they enjoy sexual contacts with them. It behooves parents to explain to their youngsters that those feelings or behaviors do not necessarily signify homosexuality or bisexuality, that are shared by a large number of teenagers, and that in most cases, they disappear later in life.

IS THERE ANY FOOLPROOF WAY TO PREVENT PREGNANCY?

The only foolproof pregnancy prevention is sexual abstinence (refraining from sexual intercourse).

WHAT ABOUT OTHER METHODS OF CONTRACEPTION?

Contraceptive methods such as condoms, the pill, subcutaneous pellets of female hormones, vaginal spermicides, an intrauterine device, and others may reduce the chances of pregnancy, but they do not provide a 100% guarantee. In cases of inability or unwillingness to be abstinent, the proper use of a non-defective condom may help in preventing pregnancy and the transmission of some serious sexually transmitted diseases (STDs).

The least effective methods of pregnancy prevention are the withdrawal technique of pulling the penis out of the vagina just before the male's orgasm and ejaculation and the rhythm method, or calculation of the female's ovulation period in what is often an irregular menstrual cycle. The risks of those methods should be obvious.

ISN'T SEXUAL ABSTINENCE OBSOLETE NOWADAYS?

Far from being obsolete, sexual abstinence is a noble and valued practice. Despite being hard to stick to in our increasingly liberal world, it offers many definitive advantages such as the prevention of STDs, unwanted pregnancy, and all of their potentially serious consequences.

Unfortunately, early sexual activity is practiced by over two-thirds of teenagers in the United States and some European countries. It is usually provoked by factors such as peer pressure, seeking proof of attractiveness, imitation, curiosity, stress, loneliness, fear of social isolation, desire to make new friends, and apprehension of losing a boyfriend or girlfriend by refusing sexual contact.

WHAT ARE THE CONCERNS ABOUT EARLY SEXUAL ACTIVITY?

Most youngsters who engage in sex are not ready for sexual intimacy or its aftermath. They feel untouchable by STDs, ignore or refuse any preventive measures, and are not emotionally mature enough to assume responsibility for their acts. Some, especially those abusing drugs or alcohol, may be unable to control themselves; under these circumstances, some boys may not accept a girl's no during a sexual encounter as a definite no to be respected, with grave or even catastrophic consequences.

Adolescents should discard the pervasive notions that for boys, no sex means no love, and that for girls, no love means no sex. Instead, they should be encouraged to accept the simple fact that couples can express affection and love, and derive pleasure, in so many different ways—kissing, hugging, caressing, holding hands, enjoying a long walk, listening to music, dancing—without having sex.

Adolescents need their parents' guidance, support, and assistance to understand sexual feelings, define proper sexual behavior, respect others, and conduct themselves with dignity. They have to understand that they do not need to engage in multiple sexual contacts with numerous partners to prove their virility, manhood, or sexual prowess, while increasing their risk of contracting (and transmitting) serious STDs such as AIDS, gonorrhea, syphilis, and hepatitis.

It has been proven that when youngsters acquire social skills with the assistance of effective, evidence-based programs designed and applied by educators or parents, they are less likely to engage in unprotected sexual practices, suffer from STDs, or have an unwanted pregnancy.

As for the common argument that boys and girls need to acquire sexual experience early on to be better lovers later in life, allow me to disagree with this erroneous belief (which is unfortunately supported by some so-called sex experts). It is greatly preferable for our teenage boys and girls to wait to acquire such experiences until adulthood, when they are mature and responsible enough to engage in intelligent, clean, and healthy sexual intimacy.

WHAT IS NONVOLITIONAL SEX?

In simple terms, *nonvolitional sex* usually means that someone is forced to have sex against his or her will. This abhorrent, immoral, dirty behavior violates a person's basic right to choose willingly whether to engage in sexual activity, with whom, and in what way (Kalmuss D 2004).

The spectrum of nonvolitional sex includes rape, sexual abuse of children, sexual violence against prostitutes or against people with nonconventional sexual identities, sex trafficking, and any other form of forced sexual activity. It is a criminal act to be condemned in the strongest terms and given the stiffest legal punishment as a deterrent.

Volitional sex and sexual health are basic human rights to be fully respected. All sex education should clearly establish a rigid prohibition against nonvolitional sex. Educators and parents should stress to children and teenagers that nonvolitional sex threatens physical and mental health and may have dire consequences for both participants.

Principles to be taught—and lived—include advocacy for sexual rights, the importance of assuming full responsibility for one's sexual behavior, gender equality, and tolerance for persons with nonconventional sexual identities. Comprehensive, sound sex education programs are of utmost importance in instilling healthy values and defining appropriate sexual behavior.

WHAT ARE THE HEALTH BENEFITS OF SEX?

Although the medical literature is studded with information and warnings regarding sexual expression, unfortunately, few articles are related to the health benefits of sexual expression. Several presentations at the First World Congress for Sexual Health, which was held in Sydney, Australia, on April 15–19, 2007, by Drs. W. Gianotten, B. Whipple, and T. Hull, stressed the benefits of sexuality on physical, reproductive, social, and emotional health. Sexual expression was found to have a positive effect on decreased mortality, lower incidence of fatal coronary artery disease, and lower risk of breast cancer in women and prostatic cancer in men. It also positively influences conception and pregnancy, and it decreases the incidence of preeclampsia and preterm delivery. Among its other benefits, an increase in testosterone levels before and after sexual activity may contribute to the prevention of heart attacks; prove a bolster to the immune system; aid in longevity, especially for women; and serve as a boost to general well-being and the quality of life and relationships. A well-known joke relates to an angry man who shouts at his wife, who repeatedly refuses to have sexual intercourse with him, "You are really trying to kill me!" According to the latest research, this may actually be true.

Chapter Three

MALE ANATOMY

God gave me a brain and a penis, and enough blood to run one at a time.
Robin Williams

The penis has been dubbed "the barometer of a man's health," and rightly so, as any abnormality in its anatomy, physiology, or functioning may reflect an underlying disease or disorder. Furthermore, the penis is considered to be the symbol of virility, power, manhood, strength, and authority. This explains the obsession of many men with the size of their penises. In an Internet-based survey of 52,031 heterosexual men, 66% rated their penises as average, 22% as large, and 12% as small (Lever J et al. 2006). Unfortunately, despite the seeming obsession with this vital organ among the majority of men (and quite a few women), most people are ignorant of even the basics of penile function and dysfunction. Here are answers to several frequently asked questions—and perhaps to some you've been unable to ask.

WHAT IS THE NORMAL LENGTH AND CIRCUMFERENCE OF THE ADULT PENIS?

No so-called normal penis size can be universally applied. Penile dimensions differ according to heredity, race, amount of suprapubic fat, age, and serum testosterone level, and even vary from one country to another.

The medical literature reports that the average length of the healthy adult penis in the United States is 3.5 inches (8.8 cm) when flaccid, about 4.9 inches (12.4 cm) when stretched, and 5.1 inches (12.9 cm) when erect; the average flaccid girth is 3.7 inches (9.4 cm) (Wessells H et al. 1996b). Other reported measurements (Chen J et al. 2000; Ponchietti R et al. 2001; Schneider T et al. 2001; Harding R, Colombok SE 2002; Son H et al. 2003; Syropoulos E et al. 2003; Awwad Z et al. 2005) from various countries follow:

> Average flaccid length is 3.72 inches for Jordanians, 3.6 inches for Italians, and 2.76 inches for Koreans, and among Germans, 3.68 inches for ages 18–19 and 3.44 inches for ages 40–68.
> Average stretched length is 5.4 inches for Jordanians, 4.87 inches for Greeks, 5.2–6.12 inches for Britishers, 5 inches for Italians, and 3.84 inches for Koreans.
> Average erect length ranges from 5.76 inches for Germans to 6.12 inches for British gays.
> Average flaccid circumference at midshaft ranges from 3.4 inches for Koreans to 4 inches for Italians.

In general, and despite some minor international variations, the normal measurements of the penis are 3.6–4 inches for the flaccid penis, 4.6–5.2 inches for the stretched penis, and 5.6–6.4 inches for the erect penis, with a girth of 3.6–4 inches for the flaccid penis and 4.6–6 inches for the erect penis (Wylie KR, Eardley I 2007).

While the penis is flaccid, the best way to estimate its erect length is to pull back the fat pad that may be covering it, stretch the penis, and measure it from the lower edge of the pubic bone to the tip of the glans.

And before you ask, there is no correlation between the size of the penis and the size of the nose, foot, fingers, or any other body part.

HOW IMPORTANT IS PENILE SIZE TO WOMEN?

There is no shortage of controversy over this issue, especially in the lay press. Some women attribute great importance to penile size, whereas others say they do not care about it, evaluating the quality of their partners' sexual performance rather than their physical endowments. For the majority of women, it seems that quality matters more than quantity.

In a study from the Netherlands of 170 women asked about the importance of penile size in relation to sexual functioning, performance, and satisfaction, 20% rated length as important and 1% as very important, versus 55% who rated it as unimportant and 22% as totally unimportant. A similar trend emerged for penile girth, which was rated overall as more important than length (Francken AB et al. 2002). Although these findings cannot be generalized to all women worldwide, they may indicate that penile size is important to only the minority—albeit a substantial number—of women.

Unfortunately, many men equate penis size with manhood, virility, sexual power, physical attraction, and better performance. Many even seek penile lengthening, although their organ size is actually within medical norms (see the following section). A candid discussion with his sexual partner may help to alleviate a man's anxiety regarding his self-assessed "small" penis. Furthermore, the size of a small penis in its flaccid state is usually not really indicative of its erect size, as its dimensions will generally increase during erection more than those of a large flaccid penis will.

DO MEN SEEKING PENILE LENGTHENING TRULY HAVE A SMALL PENIS?

Most urologists are well aware that despite the concern manifested by many men about small penile size, the organ's size in the majority of men seeking penile augmentation is actually normal (Lee PA, Reiter EO 2002, Mondaini N et al 2002). A two-year study at the University of Florence, involving 67 men aged 16–55 who requested surgical lengthening, recently confirmed this observation. Although all of them considered their penises "short" and in need of reconstruction, none turned out to have a penis that was very short according to established norms or to suffer any other penile abnormality. About 85% of them erroneously expected a normal flaccid penis to measure 3.9 to 6.7 inches (10–17 cm); about 15% could not estimate a normal size. The majority related their misconceptions of penis size to childhood comparisons with their fathers or friends, or to later comparisons with actors in pornographic movies (Mondaini N et al. 2002).

WHAT ABOUT ALL THOSE MAGAZINE AND INTERNET ADS FOR PENILE AUGMENTATION?

Numerous quacks advertise various pills, potions, lotions, stretching devices, and operative procedures to augment the size of any penis, taking advantage of men's anxieties and desires to become more physically attractive or "sexual superheroes." Unfortunately, many men fall victim to such charlatans. In general, these methods simply and plainly do not work, despite some claims of penile lengthening of 2–4 cm with some penile extenders used for several hours daily at home but which have not been confirmed by any scientific study reported in peer-reviewed medical journals, and they can cause substantial physical and emotional harm and drain a lot of money from men's pockets without any clear benefit.

All the stretching methods are of limited efficacy because the dorsal penile nerve cannot be elongated without injury or avulsion (tearing). As mentioned in chapter 1, the advertised surgical techniques usually consist of liposuction or lipectomy of the suprapubic fat pad, cutting the sensory ligament that attaches the penis to the pubic bone, or covering the penis with skin flaps from the lower abdomen and then injecting fat to increase its girth. They produce very poor results, generally achieving a wobbling, low-hanging penis that points in any direction except the normal vertical during erection. Scarring and bumps can occur, and clumps of fat can form under the penile skin. Other potential and sometimes devastating complications include infection, ED, shortening, loss of penile sensation, persistent pain, hair growth on the penis, and urinary incontinence.

The American Urological Association, the American Society for Aesthetic Plastic Surgery, and the American Society of Plastic Surgeons have issued policy statements against cosmetic surgical augmentation of a normal-size penis. I want to emphasize as well that bigger is not always better and that quality is truly much more important than quantity. (I have, in fact, treated several men for ED who were overendowed with very large genitalia!)

WHAT COULD CAUSE A PENIS TO SHRINK?

Cold water or cold weather normally shrinks the penis, whereas warm conditions can elongate it. Psychological states such as fear, anger, and anxiety can pull the external genitalia (penis, testicles, and scrotum) closer to the body and may physiologically shorten the penis temporarily.

ARE THERE MEN WHO TRULY DO HAVE A MICROPENIS?

Cases of real micropenis, although rare, merit full evaluation and management. A suggested objective definition of a penis as abnormally short is based on proposed measurements of less than 4.5 cm for flaccid length and less than 7 cm erect or stretched (Wessells H et al. 1996b)—or, more accurately, when stretched flaccid, length is more than two standard deviations below average, according to approved norms.

A thorough medical workup for a man whose penis meets the above definition of small should include karyotyping (chromosomal examination), genetic studies, and evaluation of pituitary and testicular hormones in the bloodstream as well as testosterone and dihydrotestosterone in the genital tissue.

WHAT ARE THE MOST COMMON CAUSES OF REAL MICROPENIS?

Micropenis is a multifactorial disorder caused by genetic, hormonal, and environmental abnormalities. It can also be associated with ambiguous genitalia or malformations such as hypospadias (an abnormal location of the urethral opening) (Mondaini N, Gontero P 2005).

The essential hormones for penile growth are the androgens (male hormones) testosterone and dihydrotestosterone as well as luteinizing hormone

(LH) from the pituitary gland. In the fetus, proper penile development depends on the conversion of testosterone into dihydrotestosterone by the enzyme 5-alpha reductase in the penis, testicles, scrotum, urethra, and prostate. This development also depends on the presence of intact, functional androgen receptors in the target cells in the internal and external genitalia.

Therefore any event or abnormality that inhibits androgen production or the action of 5-alpha reductase may lead to male genital underdevelopment. Exposure of a pregnant woman to hormone-disrupting industrial and agricultural chemicals, for example, can interfere with normal sexual differentiation in the fetus. Penile underdevelopment may also result from genetic mutation of the androgen receptors or from any congenital, LH-inhibiting anomaly of the hypothalamus or pituitary gland, as LH normally stimulates the testicles' Leydig cells to secrete testosterone.

Sometimes, despite normal levels of androgens, the genital tissue is insensitive to them, with the subsequent development of a micropenis that does not respond to testosterone administration. Shortening of the penis may also occur after surgeries such as radical prostatectomy (removal of the prostate and seminal vesicles) to treat prostate cancer or after insertion of penile prostheses to manage ED. And in a few cases, no evident cause for the micropenis is detected, despite a thorough workup.

HOW IS MICROPENIS MANAGED OR TREATED?

In adults, especially in a case of the man's dissatisfaction with the size of his penis and the ensuing development of severe psychological disturbances, management of the condition depends on the diagnosed causes. Treatment may involve psychiatric counseling; education; liposuction or lipectomy of the excess suprapubic fat; hormone replacement with testosterone or LH; and penile lengthening and/or widening through valid, approved microsurgical techniques performed by a team of expert urologists and plastic surgeons.

In cases of congenital or acquired micropenis—for example, complete or partial penile severance or destruction due to accident, injury, or surgical mishap—several procedures have been effective. With myocutaneous flaps (portions of muscle and skin taken from the upper arm or lower abdomen, with preservation of the nerves), it is possible to add about 2–3 inches to the penile length, or even to create a new penis. A novel procedure using bilateral flaps of the saphenous vein to increase penile girth has also yielded encouraging results (Austoni E et al. 2002).

Even in patients with amputated penises—self-inflicted by mentally disturbed men, or suffered in an accident or at the hands of a jealous or abused wife or mistress—the majority of cases can be treated successfully by microsurgical reattachment, or alternatively, by the creation or reconstruction of a new, functional penis using grafts. More than 50 such cases have been reported in the medical literature. I've personally performed three successful microsurgical reattachments.

In cases of penile shortening postprostatectomy, daily use of a vacuum device without the constricting ring (see chapter 12) may contribute to reelongation. Other surgical techniques for penile lengthening include the Perovic procedure, which involves penile disassembly, with dissection of the glans penis off the corpora cavernosa and the insertion of a piece of the costal cartilage into the distal corpora (Perovic S et al. 2003); or subcutaneous bulking of the penis with fat, free dermal fat flaps, or biodegradable material. A recent study involving the use of a biodegradable scaffold seeded with fibroblasts configured into a tube and wrapped around the penile shaft yielded good results, with about a 3-centimeter increase in girth (Perovic SV et al. 2006).

WHAT DOES IT MEAN WHEN THE PENIS BENDS OR CURVES DURING ERECTION?

Curvature or bending of the penis ventrally (down toward the thighs), laterally (toward either side), or dorsally (back toward the body) during erection, although uncommon, may be very disturbing to the patient. It may be associated with pain, difficulty of penetration, and sometimes ED.

If a bend or curve has been present since birth, it may be due to an abnormal attachment of the penile skin or the subcutaneous fascia (tissues beneath the skin) or to abnormally short corpora cavernosa, both of which can be corrected surgically with excellent results. Ventral bending could very well be congenital and is most often linked to hypospadias (described previously). In adults, the most common cause of painful penile curvature or bending is a condition called Peyronie's disease (see chapter 7). Ventral bending, in particular, can also be acquired through a fracture of the penis (see the following section) or some other form of trauma to the genitalia.

HOW CAN A PENIS BE FRACTURED IF IT HAS NO BONE?

Application of the term *fracture* to the penis may not be fully justified, but it is accepted and used by the medical community for lack of a better description. In most of these unfortunate cases, a man with a full erection, during intercourse or even during sleep, has hit his penis on a solid object or flexed it acutely while rolling in bed. There is usually a crackling sound accompanied by pain, loss of erection, and penile swelling, with a reddish or bluish discoloration; these are due to a rupture of the tunica albuginea, seeping of blood beneath the penile skin, and development of a hematoma (a collection of clotted blood). For most, the ideal treatment is immediate surgical intervention to evacuate the leaked blood and suture the tear in the tunica. Left untreated, a penile fracture may cause scarring at the site of the rupture, with subsequent curvature of the penis during erection.

Chapter Four

RISE AND FALL: THE ERECTILE PROCESS

Sex lies at the root of life and we can never learn to reverence life until we know how to understand sex.

Havelock Ellis

The phases of the male sexual response have distinctive physiologic characteristics (Lue T et al. 2004a) that include the erectile process, which is a continuing series of neurovascular events occurring within a normal hormonal milieu (primarily, an appropriate level of serum testosterone) and with an intact psychological setup.

Translation? An erection does not occur on demand at a snap of the fingers. Several systems in the body and the mind team up to produce an erection. As described in chapter 3, the anatomy of the penis is the foundation, but erection has certain other prerequisites: an intact neurovascular system, absence of medical or psychogenic disturbance, confidence, intimacy, receptivity, excitement, and physical attraction. Physical and psychological stimulation are also required. If any of the involved mechanisms fail, an erection can become difficult or impossible to achieve or to maintain, resulting in erectile dysfunction (ED).

WHAT IS THE NORMAL MALE SEXUAL RESPONSE?

The normal human male response to sexual opportunity, as originally described by Masters and Johnson (1970), comprises five phases: desire, excitement, plateau, orgasm, and refraction, as follows:

1. A healthy and sexually functional man, who is mentally prepared for and interested in sexual activity, feels the desire to engage in lovemaking.

2. When that desire is accompanied by sexual stimulation, excitement occurs. The man becomes aroused and his penis becomes erect. Additionally, his pulse rate and blood pressure and nipple sensitivity increase, and his testicles become elevated.
3. Arousal increases and the man reaches a high plateau of sexual pleasure, associated with physiological changes such as rapid breathing, further testicular elevation and swelling, and generalized muscle relaxation. There may be a flush or even a rash over different parts of his body and a slight urethral discharge from the Cowper's glands (see the Glossary).
4. Plateau is followed by semen emission and ejaculation, together with various associated sensations perceived in his brain as pleasurable, called orgasm.
5. The final phase is the refractory period, characterized by the loss of his erection and the gradual disappearance of all other physiological signs of arousal, and during which no erection or orgasm can occur. The duration of this phase depends on such things as the man's age, the recency of his last intercourse and ejaculation, degree of subsequent sexual stimulation, and physical and psychological status.

If there are so many prerequisites for an erection, how can erections occur during sleep or in men with spinal injury or paralysis?

There are three different types of erections. A psychogenic erection is initiated by imaginative, visual, olfactory, tactile, or auditory stimulation. A reflexogenic erection, on the other hand, is produced by direct stimulation of the genitalia; this is also the type of erection that may reflexively occur in paraplegics (even though the injury, disease, or malformation of their spinal cord means that they aren't necessarily aware of, or feeling, any stimulation or erection). The third type, nocturnal erection, develops repeatedly during periods of rapid eye movement (REM) sleep, usually in the early morning period before awakening.

Nocturnal erection is something of a misnomer, as REM-related erections may also occur in a male sleeping for an extended time during the day. Erections during sleep serve as a natural physiological means to keep the cavernous tissues of the corpora well oxygenated. They occur from two to five times per night and last about 20 minutes each, usually decreasing with age in number, duration, and intensity.

Psychogenic erections differ neurologically from reflexogenic and nocturnal ones in their initiation and maintenance, but their final neurologic pathway is the same, and the vascular events in the penis are mostly similar.

IS THERE AN ON-OFF SWITCH FOR ERECTION?

Not exactly. The brain, however, is undoubtedly the most important human sex organ. In the male, the brain not only receives and processes erotic stimuli—touch, sight, sound, smell, taste, and thought—but also coordinates the steps essential for erectile development by sending messages (neural impulses) back through the nervous system to the penis.

I like to think of it this way: when a man is awake, alert, and not receiving any sexual stimulation, his brain sends constant signals to the penis not to get erect. If, for some reason, the brain stops sending these inhibitory signals, or the signals are not relayed properly by the spinal cord or other nerves, an unsolicited erection will probably occur. So the brain is the main controller that facilitates or inhibits an erection's development.

Studies taking spectroscopic MRIs during sexual excitement and erection have shown that the brain contains multiple central sex centers. The most prominent of these are located in the paraventricular medial dorsal nucleus of the thalamus and the medial preoptic nucleus of the hypothalamus. The sex centers receive, integrate, and process erotic stimuli from the body and the sensory organs. The balance between pro-erectile and antierectile stimuli in the brain sex centers determines the message or instruction that is sent back to the body via neurotransmitters.

HOW MUCH STIMULATION IS NEEDED FOR AN ERECTION?

The type and amount of erotic stimulation necessary to summon an erection varies from man to man and also with age.

Adolescent and young adult males usually have no problems obtaining erections, which may occur with (or without) minimal sexual stimulation. A healthy 18-year-old, for example, can get an erection simply by fantasy or other noncontact sexual stimuli. Young men can have two or three full sexual encounters, from erection to orgasm, in a short time with little or no foreplay required. Although progressive changes in a man's sexual response usually occur by age 30, he can still easily develop an erection during kissing or foreplay. However, after age 50, he will usually need more direct sexual stimulation to achieve a firm erection.

This gradual slowing in sexual response as the man becomes more mature and sentimental has its rewards. More often than not, the love play and the sexual relationship become more meaningful and more pleasant. In older age, a healthy man is usually able to maintain good erections but tends to require more time during foreplay to achieve one. (Note, though, that spontaneous erections occur during sleep at any age.)

I should emphasize that for any man, regardless of age, to have an erection, he generally needs an anxiety-free, relaxed atmosphere—this means no performance demands.

HOW DOES SEXUAL STIMULATION REACH THE BRAIN?

Numerous sensory receptors in the glans penis, penile skin, urethra, and corpora cavernosa—but not the corpus spongiosum—unite to form the dorsal nerve of the penis, which joins the pudendal nerve in the pelvis and perineum (the area between the base of the penis and the anus). Through the pudendal nerve, penile sensations are conveyed to an erectile center called Onuf's nucleus in the sacral spinal cord. This erectile center, in turn, transmits the neural information up to the brain's central sex centers, which are also receiving sexual/erotic stimulation from the sensory organs and the rest of the body. As previously noted, the balance between pro-erectile and antierectile stimuli in the brain's sex centers determines whether or not an erection will result.

HOW DOES THE BRAIN THEN INFLUENCE THE BODY'S RESPONSE?

When a healthy man is aroused by erotic stimuli and the pro-erectile stimuli are sufficient for his brain's sex centers to initiate the development of an erection, the sex centers release the neurotransmitters dopamine and oxytocin. These overcome the antierectile effect of the neurotransmitters noradrenaline and serotonin, thereby inhibiting the sympathetic nervous system's usual vasoconstrictive action on the penile arteries (Lue T et al. 2004a). Dopamine and oxytocin further activate Onuf's nucleus, the sacral spinal cord's erectile center.

From there, parasympathetic nerves convey the neural impulses down to the penis via the cavernous nerves, causing the release of additional chemicals that are actively involved in producing an erection through penile vasodilation. Additional parasympathetic stimulation down through the pudendal nerve causes the ischiocavernous muscles surrounding the corpora cavernosa to contract, increasing the rigidity of the erection. The pudendal nerve also conveys sensations of sexual pleasure and orgasm from the penis back up to the brain.

In a reflexogenic erection, however, the process is somewhat different. Direct sexual stimulation sends neural impulses up through the penile dorsal nerve to the spinal erectile center; from there, stimulation travels back down to the penis via the parasympathetic and cavernous nerves, without being modulated by the brain.

WHAT DO THE NERVES AND CHEMICALS HAVE TO DO WITH BLOOD FLOW TO THE PENIS?

Neurobiochemical processes at the molecular level underlie the physiology of erection. During sexual arousal, the previously described parasympathetic nerve stimulation to the penile tissue causes the release of neurotransmitters and other chemicals from the nerve terminals and the vascular endothelium (the lining of the arteries and sinuses) in the penis. These chemicals cause smooth muscle relaxation and dilation of the cavernous blood vessels and their tributaries, the helicine arteries, which supply blood to the vascular sinuses in the corpora cavernosa. The synchronized widening of these vessels and sinuses produces tumescence by increasing blood flow to the penis.

Within the corpora, the endings of nonadrenergic/noncholinergic nerves secrete the neurotransmitters acetylcholine and nitric oxide (NO). NO may also be released from the vascular endothelium. NO is produced in the body by the action of the enzyme nitric oxide synthase on the substance L-arginine in the presence of adequate dihydrotestosterone. NO is the chemical considered to be principally responsible for the vascular dilation in erection. It may also be involved in storing and propagating neural impulses in the spinal cord and the pelvic nerves.

It seems that the oxygen content of the penile tissues and the level of testosterone in the bloodstream also significantly affect the secretion of NO. Therefore any obstruction of the penile vessels that precludes normal delivery of oxygenated blood to the penile tissue may impair the secretion of NO and lead to ED (see chapter 7).

NO penetrates the smooth muscle cells in the walls of the penile arteries and sinuses, where it stimulates the enzyme guanylate cyclase to convert the naturally occurring compound guanosine triphosphate into another substance required for erection, cyclic guanosine monophosphate (cGMP). A potent smooth muscle relaxant and vasodilator, cGMP relaxes the vessels by lowering the amount of calcium inside their muscle cells to reduce the muscle tone.

With the resulting dilation of the penile vessels, blood flows rapidly into the penis at high volume and progressively increasing pressure. This pressure may exceed the systolic pressure (blood pressure during heart contractions) in the rest of the body's peripheral arteries. The cavernous tissues become engorged with blood, which stays in the penis because the penile veins are compressed, and with the accompanying contraction of the penile muscles, erection is achieved and maintained (see following section).

Additional substances, including vasoactive intestinal peptide (VIP), calcitonin gene-related peptide, adenosine, cyclic adenosine monophosphate, adenosine triphosphate, and prostaglandin E1, have been reported to be involved in the erectile process as well. Others may yet be identified; for example, it was recently discovered that activation of calcium-sensitizing pathways contributes to penile flaccidity, whereas their deactivation contributes to erection.

WOULDN'T IT BE SIMPLER IF THE PENILE ARTERIES WERE ALWAYS WIDE OPEN?

If this were the case, the penis would be in a constant state of erection. This could be quite painful, not to mention embarrassing and potentially dangerous.

HOW DOES INCREASED BLOOD FLOW MAKE THE PENIS ERECT?

Prior to arousal, when the penis is totally flaccid and its arteries and sinuses are contracted, penile blood flow is low, amounting to about 1–2 milliliters per minute, but when sexual stimulation and excitement produce penile vasodilation, penile blood flow increases to about 90 milliliters per minute.

This increased inflow to the corpora swells the penis, which becomes tumescent: longer and thicker but not yet hard. Then, as more blood flows into the penis and the corpora (mainly, the cavernosa) become engorged, the dilated penile sinuses crowd and compress the veins of the penis against the tunica albuginea. This compression dramatically reduces the penile venous outflow, trapping blood within the penis.

With more blood coming in than going out, pressure in the penis builds, pushing in all directions—much like an inflating balloon—and as a result of this pressure the congested penis straightens, elongates, expands, and becomes firmly erect. Once the penis is full to capacity, blood flow both in and out of the corpora decreases to a minimum and then stops completely after the ischiocavernous muscles contract, maintaining a rigid erection (see Figure 4.1).

Figure 4.1
Mechanism of the Erectile Process

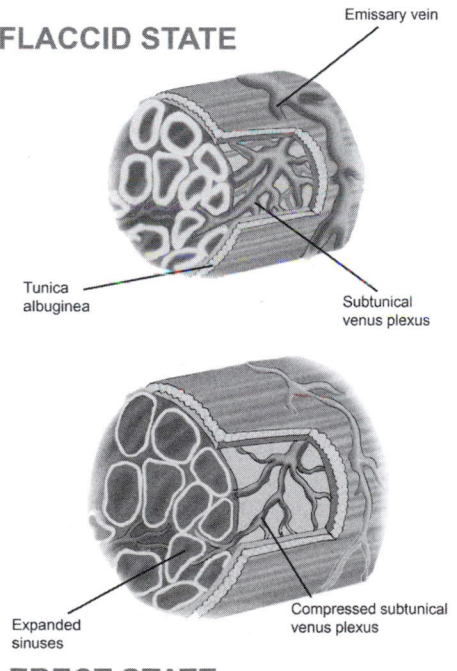

Courtesy of Alexander Balmaceda.

DOES A MAN DEVELOP AN ERECTION EVERY TIME HIS PENILE ARTERIES EXPAND?

In principle, yes, with a major qualification: his arteries must be healthy, and there must be no abnormal leakage of blood from the penis through the veins. As detailed previously, erection is produced not only by increased penile arterial blood flow, but also by decreased penile venous outflow. (If this outflow decreases too much for too long, an overly prolonged erection, or priapism, may pose a serious problem.)

WHAT IS THE NORMAL DURATION OF ERECTION BEFORE EJACULATION?

The length of time a man is able to maintain an erection is an important facet of his normal sexual functioning. Most young men can maintain a firm erection for at least 5–15 minutes, and some individuals for more than half an hour. On average, after penetration, most men can sustain their erection for about 8–10 minutes before ejaculation. The number of orgasms experienced successively during intercourse also varies from man to man. Most are satisfied with one orgasm per sexual encounter, but others need several for total satisfaction. Medically speaking, and in the absence of any sexual dysfunction, all of these men are so-called normal.

WHAT BRINGS ABOUT THE END OF AN ERECTION?

After orgasm and ejaculation, or when erotic physical and psychological stimulation ceases, the penile arteries and sinuses narrow to their normal diameter, the veins are decompressed, and the unimpeded outflow of blood from the penis leads to the loss of the erection and the return of flaccidity.

As detailed previously, dilation of the penile arteries and vascular sinuses is principally controlled by the nitrergic system, based on the secretion of neurotransmitters and vasodilators (NO, acetylcholine, cGMP, and such) from the parasympathetic nervous system and the vessels' lining. By contrast, constriction of the penile arteries and sinuses is principally controlled by the vipergenic system, which relies on VIP, on secretion of the vasoconstrictive hormones adrenalin and noradrenalin from the sympathetic nervous system, and on beta-2 adrenergic receptors to keep the penile vessels and sinuses partially closed.

Other substances called endothelins, secreted by the vessels' lining, may also contribute to constriction of the penile vessels. Chemicals such as prostaglandin F2a, prostanoids, and angiotensin II are involved as well. These vasoconstrictive substances restore the normal resistance to increased blood flow in the penile arteries and sinuses, preventing the occurrence of a subsequent erection for the duration of the refractory period. As previously noted, this period lasts from a few minutes to several hours, according to the man's age and other factors.

Activity of VIP, endothelins, and norepinephrine, in fact, may underlie psychogenic ED, as they contract the penile arteries and sinuses in response to stress, anxiety, and other psychological or emotional factors (see chapter 8).

WHAT HAPPENS IF BLOOD STAYS TRAPPED IN THE PENIS AND THE ERECTION PERSISTS?

A persistent, possibly painful erection not associated with ongoing sexual desire or pleasure is called priapism. It can last for more than four hours and may cause penile damage if left untreated.

For appropriate treatment, it is important to determine whether the condition is low-flow or high-flow priapism. Of the two, the low-flow or ischemic type, due to entrapment of blood in the corpora cavernosa with reduced outflow of blood through the veins, is more common. Intracorporeal injection of vasodilators (see chapter 12) is the most frequent cause of low-flow priapism. Other causes follow:

- Conditions that lead to slowing and sludging of blood in the penile vascular sinuses (e.g., hematologic diseases such as sickle cell anemia, leukemia, multiple myeloma, thrombophelia, polycythemia, or thalassemia)
- Certain antihypertensive, antipsychotic, anticoagulant, and recreational drugs
- Certain neurologic conditions
- Trauma to the perineum from straddle injury or cycling
- Locally invasive or metastatic cancer (such as from the bladder, prostate, urethra, lung, or kidney) involving the penis

In some cases, even a thorough evaluation cannot identify the priapism's etiology.

When it is the low-flow type, Doppler ultrasonography shows no blood flow inside the penile vasculature, and analysis of a sample of the dark blood drawn from the corpora reveals low oxygen content with acidosis (accumulation of acid). Untreated, this emergency condition can result in poor oxygenation of the penile tissue, cell death, and severe scarring.

Management of low-flow priapism depends on its duration, etiology (if known), and symptom severity. The initial measures—which are usually not very successful—include ice packs, sedatives, analgesics (for pain), intranasal oxygen, and oral terbutaline (a vasoconstrictor). The next steps, if needed, are aspiration of blood from the corpora; intracorporeal injection of vasoconstrictors such as phenylephrine, epinephrine, or aramine; and/or manual compression of the penis for several minutes, which may yield good results. If these fail, or if the priapism recurs after a period of detumescence, one of several surgical techniques is used to shunt blood from the affected corpus cavernosum to the corpus spongiosum (which is not involved in the pathology) or to the saphenous vein in the upper leg.

High-flow priapism usually results from blunt trauma to the penis or perineum. In these cases, the abnormal erection is typically softer and nonpainful; the aspirated blood is bright red, well oxygenated, and nonacidotic; and Doppler ultrasonography shows adequate penile blood flow. High-flow priapism does not require emergency measures and may subside spontaneously without treatment or simply with manual compression of the penis. But if it persists, embolization (occlusion by scarring solutions or coils) or surgical ligation (tying off) of the bleeding penile vessel can be performed, with excellent results.

Stuttering priapism is a term for low-flow priapism's frequent recurrence after initially successful therapy. Several oral medications, such as bicalutamide, baclofen, ketokonazole, flutamide, gonadotropin releasing hormone (GnRH) agonists (which mimic the action of GnRH), and digoxin, have been effective in preventing stuttering priapism. Recently, two of the phosphodiesterase type 5 inhibitors (Viagra and Cialis; see chapter 11) have also been used successfully for this purpose. In rare cases that don't respond to conservative nonsurgical measures, the patient may be instructed to inject his penis with a vasoconstricting substance whenever a prolonged involuntary erection occurs, or he may require a surgical shunt, as described previously.

If ED develops secondary to priapism or surgery for priapism, a penile prosthesis can be inserted (see chapter 13).

Chapter Five

A TRAGEDY OF THE BEDROOM: SEXUAL DYSFUNCTION

> There exist fundamental rights for the individual, including the right to sexual health and a capacity to enjoy and control sexual and reproductive behavior in accordance with a social personal ethic.
>
> World Health Organization Guidelines

Understanding normal sexual function is necessary for understanding sexual dysfunction. To that end, the preceding chapters detailed the male sexual response at anatomical, physiological, and neurobiochemical levels. As described, erection relies on healthy vascular and neurologic tissue and genital organs as well as an adequate male hormonal milieu. Numerous factors pertaining to the brain, spinal cord, nerves, blood vessels, smooth muscles, and hormones are crucial to a man's optimal sexual expression and pleasure.

But there is, of course, much more to sex than a man's ability to have an erection. Sexual functioning is a complex process that depends on age, genetic traits, character, life experience, physical capacity, sexual impulses, fantasies, inhibitions, sentiments, ideals, and motivation. Personality, attitudes toward sexuality, and past sexual experiences as well as cultural, familial, religious, and social influences contribute significantly to the character and composition of an individual's sexual relationships. The interaction and relationship between the partners is of primary importance to sexual functioning and enjoyment.

Unfortunately, millions of men, for physical and/or psychological reasons, have lost interest in sex, cannot achieve an erection, or cannot sustain one. Fortunately, sexual dysfunction need not be permanent; once identified, it can be managed, and the sufferer can once again experience the joys of the sexual response and a sexual relationship. This chapter attempts to clarify misconceptions about male sexual dysfunction, in general, and erectile dysfunction (ED), in particular. Knowledge and understanding eases anxiety and confusion about these problems, enables objective and positive discussion, and is a vital first step toward treatment.

SEX: ART AND CONTINUING EXPERIENCE

The majority of people usually engage in sexual activities that fall in the midrange between extremes. It is important to realize that so-called uncommon sexual behaviors or changes in a usual sexual pattern are not necessarily abnormal. Even those individuals whose behavior is either of two extremes—such as very frequent sexual encounters, or very rare encounters, for example—do not necessarily have reason for concern. (An individual who cannot accept the status of his or her sex life, however, for whatever reason, should consider seeking professional help.)

Almost all men occasionally experience episodes of sexual inadequacy that are usually of no consequence or importance. Normal men may experience a very strong sexual desire but without an erection, or sometimes an erection and even ejaculation without any sexual stimulation. These occasional anomalies may occur in times of marked anxiety, anger, or nervousness. Changes in an individual's or couple's standard sexual behavior may occur in an especially encouraging or facilitating situation such as a honeymoon, vacation, or romantic weekend, or conversely, in an especially discouraging or off-putting situation such as an illness, financial crisis, or other time of stress.

It must be emphasized that erection and intercourse cannot be standardized. Cultural, ethnic, social, and personal factors influence the ways different men perceive their sexual potency. To many men, the quality, staying power, frequency, and/or number of successive erections are defining characteristics. For instance, a man who is accustomed to achieving daily erections lasting 15 minutes or more may feel impotent if his frequency of erections decreases to two or three per week or if his erection lasts only about five minutes. But another man may feel completely potent if he has erections once or twice a week lasting four to five minutes.

Generally speaking, young couples in today's world have sexual intercourse an average of two or three times a week—which means that many couples have sex more often than that and many have it less. Every couple differs in the time required for full sexual satisfaction; even separate episodes with the same sexual partner may vary in the time required. What one couple considers normal sexual functioning and behavior may be considered abnormal by another. Ultimately, a man's potency is best gauged by the sexual satisfaction of both partners, not just by penis size, frequency or duration of erections or intercourse, or amount of time involved.

For a specific example of the continuum of normal, consider the changes in sexual response and function that occur naturally with age. As noted in chapter 4, the achievement and maintenance of erections may become inconsistent later in a man's life and normally require more direct genital stimulation. An older man generally notices that his penile sensitivity decreases, erections are softer, orgasms are less intense, ejaculation is less forceful, and there is less volume of ejaculate (or none at all); following ejaculation, it may be several hours or even days before he can get another erection. His physiological (and emotional) need for orgasm decreases as he gets older, and his frequency of sexual intercourse usually decreases as well, to an average of less than once a month by age 75. Nevertheless, a man can enjoy so-called normal sex, regardless of his age, as long as his physical and psychological health and his interrelational circumstances allow.

A recent survey of 1,185 men aged 20–79 from Norway and the United States found, as might be expected, greater incidences of both ED and reduced sexual desire in older men. However, the men in their fifties reported similar satisfaction with their sex lives to the men in their twenties, and satisfaction greater than that was reported by the men in their thirties and forties, despite the fact that they also reported decreased sex drive and erectile and ejaculatory quality with advancing age. Analysis showed that age accounted for 22% of the variance in sex drive and 33% and 23% of the variances in erectile and ejaculatory issues, respectively, but only accounted for 3% of the variance in sexual satisfaction (Mykletun A et al. 2006).

What those results really mean is that men in their fifties and older may experience more problems with erection and ejaculation, but these problems do not seem to lessen their overall sexual satisfaction. According to psychologist Dr. Bracey, such findings are not surprising. In a British Broadcasting Corporation interview (February 21, 2006), he suggested that men in their thirties and forties may be too stressed by other things in life (such as career) to be able to fully enjoy sex, whereas men in their fifties, who may have "adjusted to what they want out of life and tend to be less hung up," may be able to derive more pleasure from sex in their maturity.

Nowadays, to be a good lover requires adequate technical ability and lack of emotional inhibition. Beyond the body contact, fondling, and various sexual maneuvers lie the impulses, emotions, sentiments, and fantasies that shape the sexual relationship, which is an encounter between two bodies, two subconsciouses, two minds, and two desires. It is a repeated experience and adventure that can be highly satisfying, but sometimes threatening, as it may reveal our fragility (Salvi FM 2006). According to certain psychologists, sexuality represents a subconscious desire to experience again the pleasurable sensations experienced during childhood that were provided by the mother, with her affectionate and gentle touching and fondling of our body. A sexual relationship implies physical and emotional sharing between two persons, with the intent of providing mutual pleasure and not using the sexual partner as a sex object for selfish gratification. Sex is a unique experience, which may involve affection, satisfaction, fear, desire, intimacy, inhibition, invention, fantasy, and improvisation. It is an encounter of two bodies, two minds, and two souls trying to explore each other and to provide the ultimate mutual physical pleasure. The art of sex involves reaching beyond the pleasure of orgasm by learning how to relax, how to breathe deeply, how to manage and nurture our body, and how to free our sexual instinct from any restriction and inhibition. It also involves the desire to learn and progress sexually, to experiment with the discovery of new fantasies and experiences, and to establish a relationship that reaches beyond the physical contact to include love, sharing, and deep knowledge of our bodies and that of our partners. Sexuality as a Tantra, a tradition experienced for over a thousand years, may lead to ecstasy when the pleasure of the body combines with the pleasure of the heart and mind to reach the universal cosmic conscience.

The tragedy of sexual failure is a devastating experience, especially for men; it may affect their sense of virility, manhood, self-respect, and pride at any age and expose the man to emotional and psychological disturbances. It may open the gates of hell for millions of men, as we will see later in the book.

NOT JUST FOR MEN

Sexual dysfunctions do not only afflict men. Women also experience them in the form of lack of interest in sex, low desire, poor arousal, frigidity, absence of vaginal lubrication, orgasmic inhibition, and pain during coitus. At times, sexual dysfunction may be present in both partners in a relationship.

IMPOTENCE, SEXUAL DYSFUNCTION, ERECTILE DYSFUNCTION (ED): WHAT DOES IT ALL MEAN?

Many people do not like the term *impotence* because of its negative connotation. It is also rather vague and imprecise, which is one of the reasons it has been largely replaced by other terms in the medical literature. In common parlance, *erectile dysfunction* is often used as a synonym for *impotence*, but the two terms are not actually interchangeable, as one is more strictly an erectile failure than the other. Furthermore, neither term adequately characterizes the full range of male sexual disturbances. *Sexual dysfunction* is a broader term that encompasses ejaculatory problems, lack of orgasm, decreased libido, ED, and other conditions that preclude normal sexual functioning or satisfaction.

For practical purposes, I define a potent (sexually functional) man as one who has a high level of desire and is able, for a majority of his sexual encounters, to achieve an erection of sufficient quality to permit penetration, intercourse, orgasm, and ejaculation. He should be able to maintain his erection for at least the minimum time necessary to satisfy both partners. Conversely, I consider a man who cannot develop an erection of sufficient rigidity or duration for intercourse to the full satisfaction of both parties to be sexually dysfunctional; more precisely, he is suffering from ED. Beyond this, there is no single standard or average that can—or should—be applied.

Classifying Male Sexual Dysfunction

The most common male sexual dysfunctions are (1) ED, (2) premature ejaculation, (3) retarded or absent ejaculation, (4) inhibited sexual desire or drive, (5) absence of orgasm, and (6) deviations and perversions. Sexual dysfunction may be primary, which means that it has persisted for all of a person's life (though it may not have been apparent until he or she became sexually active), or secondary, which means that a person who previously functioned well, sexually speaking, subsequently developed the dysfunction.

ED

ED is the inability of a male to achieve or to maintain an erection of adequate quality and duration to permit satisfactory sexual performance and sexual gratification. It can occur in a man whose libido (sex drive) is intact (and therefore unfulfilled), or it can be associated with decreased or absent sex drive. ED is not a disease per se, but rather the clinical manifestation of one or more organic and/or psychogenic conditions. ED is not necessarily an all-or-none problem; rather, it is usually a matter of degree, ranging from minor to complete. It cuts across race, nationality, and socioeconomic factors; occurs at all ages; and varies in severity and duration from man to man. Almost all married men experience occasional episodes of ED.

Some "sexperts" contend that a man should fail in at least 50% of his sexual encounters before he is considered to have ED, but they would get an argument from men who are unsuccessful 99% of the time and would see 50% as a vast improvement. Others say that a minimum of five minutes of erection firm enough for intercourse denotes normal erectile function, but they would also get an argument, especially from men who cannot maintain an erection for 15 minutes or more—these men, though far from "impotent," are disappointed with their sexual function and may consider themselves to have ED, however illogical that may seem to others.

Patterns of ED differ among men. Some men lose their erections when they get anxious; some can achieve erections only during foreplay; others may gain an erection only to lose it at the moment of penetration or during intercourse. Some men may have erections through masturbation, or only in deviant situations (e.g., with pornography or during unusual sexual encounters), but fail to achieve or maintain erections under normal circumstances or with their primary sexual partner—such a man is anatomically potent, but psychologically, he has ED.

The International Society of Impotence Research (Lizza EF, Rosen RC 1999) and the American Urological Association's treatment guidelines (Montague DK et al. 2005) have both classified ED into five categories: (1) vasculogenic (arterial, cavernosal, and mixed), (2) psychogenic (situational and generalized), (3) neurogenic, (4) endocrinologic, and (5) drug induced. The etiologies, treatments, and therapeutic outcomes are different for each of these five categories as well as for primary versus secondary ED.

The prognosis for a man with ED depends on the condition's duration, the underlying cause(s), the man's willingness to seek medical advice and accept treatment, and the presence of aggravating conditions such as obesity, heavy smoking, lack of exercise, chronic alcoholism, drug addiction, unacknowledged homosexuality, or sexual deviations. Additional physical and psychological factors can also influence therapeutic success.

Mind and Body

For the purpose of organizing a large body of material, this book roughly divides the physical and psychological causes of ED (chapters 7 and 8). But when it comes to ED, strict etiologic classification between organic and psychogenic is an oversimplification. ED is a multifaceted condition, and its etiology is often multifactorial. The various predisposing and contributing factors run the gamut from age, chronic health conditions, and emotional disorders to obesity, lack of exercise, and the use of certain medications and other substances. Any organic or psychological disorder that affects the brain, nervous system, vascular system, endocrine system, or genitourinary system—or, even more specifically, affects any part of the penis—can lead to a man's inability to develop or maintain a firm erection for a period long enough for successful sexual intercourse.

Before 1980, most primary ED was considered to be psychogenic. Newer studies, however, have demonstrated that organic causes play a role in the majority of primary ED cases and that many cases—up to about 45%—involve a combination of physical and psychological factors. Recent advances in diagnostic sophistication and our understanding of erection have shown that for ED overall (primary and secondary combined), causes are purely organic or mixed in 70% to 90% and psychogenic in about 10% to 25%, according to age. In general, about 75% of ED cases in men younger than 40 are psychogenic or combined; by comparison, about 75% of ED cases in men over 60 are organic. Irrespective of its cause, most patients with ED experience emotional reactions to it—this is a natural response to what can be a devastating problem. Male sexual dysfunction can even result in psychological disturbances requiring evaluation and treatment.

Prevalence and Epidemiology

In the United States alone, ED affects about 15–30 million men. About 48% of the American male population over the age of 50 may suffer from ED, with the incidence increasing with age to reach about 75% in men 70 or older. Recent statistics for American men include the following:

- A study of 2,115 men aged 40–79 revealed an overall incidence of severe ED (infrequent or no erections) of about 12%, ranging from 1% in young men to about 25% in the oldest group. (Panser LA et al. 1995)
- Longitudinal results from the 1987–1989 Massachusetts Male Aging Study (MMAS) revealed that in 1,700 men aged 40–70, the combined prevalence of minimal, moderate, and severe ED was 52%. ED's combined prevalence was also shown to increase with age, affecting about 40% of men aged 40–49 and almost 70% of those aged 70–79. Comparing age 40 to age 70, the prevalence of severe ED rose from about 5% to about 15%, moderate ED doubled from 17% to 34%, and minimal ED held constant at 17%. An update of the MMAS showed a twofold increase in ED with each decade of life. (Feldman HA et al. 1994; Johannes CB et al. 2000)

Accurate figures for ED's global incidence are difficult to obtain, partly because the discussion of sex is still taboo in several parts of the world. Many men deny any experience of sexual inadequacy out of embarrassment or ignorance; others simply consider it a natural, inevitable consequence of old age and don't give it another thought. International statistics include the following:

- In Germany, the Cologne Male Study revealed a 19.2% prevalence of ED among 4,489 men aged 30–80. (Braun M et al. 2000)
- Carson et al. (2006) found that over 50% of men aged 40–70 had ED of different degrees, with about 10% complaining of complete ED, about 25% of moderate ED, and 17% of minimal ED. Furthermore, of 500 men who visited urologists for urinary symptoms unrelated to ED, about 44% had ED, and yet about 74% of those men did not discuss it with any physician out of embarrassment.
- A study of 1,688 elderly Dutch men found that significant ED, with severely reduced rigidity or no erections, was reported in 3% of men aged 50 to 54 and 26% of men aged 70 to 78. The prevalence of severely reduced or absent ejaculatory volume also increased from 3% to 35% in those age groups. (Blanker MH et al. 2001)

- A systematic review of the prevalence of ED based on 23 studies from Europe, the United States, Asia, and Australia revealed that the prevalence of ED ranged from 2% in men younger than 40 to 86% in men over the age of 80. (Prins J et al. 2002)
- Several studies involving different countries and including men aged 18–90 were reported at the Second International Consultation on Sexual Dysfunctions in 2003, with high rates of ED worldwide that increased with each decade of life. Overall, the prevalence of ED was 1% to 9% for men aged 18–39, 3% to 15% for men aged 40–49, 2% to 35% for men aged 50–59, 11% to 49% for men aged 60–69, and 22% to 79% for men aged 70 and older. (Althof SE et al. 2003; Basson R et al. 2003; Bondil P et al. 2003; McMahon CG, Meston C 2003; Meyer KF et al. 2003)
- Twenty-three worldwide studies using the Sexual Health Inventory for Men (SHIM) revealed ED prevalences of 64% in Leon, Spain; 56% in West Virginia; 54% in Porto Allegre, Brazil; and 32% in Japan. (Cappelleri JC, Rosen RC 2005)

It is estimated that in total, about 150 million men worldwide suffer from some degree of ED, and it is projected that this number will double by the year 2025, as the male population becomes increasingly older. These figures, however, doubtless underestimate the true global prevalence of ED.

Chapter Six

EFFECTS OF SEXUAL DYSFUNCTION ON MEN AND THEIR PARTNERS

There is no such a thing as an uninvolved partner in a marriage where sexual dysfunction exists.

William Masters and Virginia Johnson

Sex is an integral part of an intimate relationship and forms the basis for a couple's shared love and respect, but many people cannot fully enjoy these pleasures. A sexually dysfunctional man, for example, may lack the desire or self-confidence to participate in sexual activity. He may not be able to focus his attention on arousal activities. He may ejaculate prematurely, or lose his erection before his sexual partner is sexually satisfied, or he may develop and maintain an erection for a long time but without being able to reach orgasm or ejaculate.

Other men with sexual dysfunction may find that they cannot achieve an erection of sufficient rigidity for intercourse—or cannot get an erection at all. They may be too anxious during the sexual act. They may be ignorant of various sexual techniques. They may not indulge in adequate or proper foreplay and lack adequate sexual stimulation. They may not experience appropriate or enjoyable mental or emotional attitudes as they become sexually aroused.

Sexual dysfunction can destroy a marital or other sexual relationship. Understanding this affliction, how it affects the sufferer's and others' lives, and how the sufferer can free himself or herself is essential for the maintenance and preservation of any current or future sexual relationship.

THE EMOTIONAL IMPACT OF SEXUAL DYSFUNCTION

Consider a scandal that rocked American society in 1937. Some readers may still remember the stunning beauty of movie star Jean Harlow, the first Hollywood "sex goddess." At the age of 21, she married 40-year-old producer Paul Bern, but their wedding night proved disastrous when she realized that Bern was "underendowed" and probably impotent. Her agent later reported that Harlow was then beaten ferociously with a cane by her humiliated husband, sustaining several broken bones. Perhaps Bern had believed that by marrying a young woman with tremendous sex appeal, he could overcome his sexual inadequacy—and when this failed, he became violent and inflicted physical punishment on her. Despite the couple's public reconciliation and manifestations of affection, their relationship was in shambles. When Bern once tried to impress her by "wearing a contraption designed to make the most of his meager assets she felt disgusted." Two months after their wedding, Bern committed suicide by shooting himself in the head, leaving a note: "Dearest dear: Unfortunately this is the only way to make good the frightful wrong I have done you and to wipe my frightful humiliation. I love you. Paul" (Blundell N 1994, 137). This particularly dramatic example illustrates the potentially devastating effects of sexual dysfunction on the individual and the couple.

It is often said that a man can stoically confront wars, hurricanes, tornados, earthquakes, diseases, and other tragedies with great courage and determination, but when he can't function sexually as he wishes, he may feel devastated, depressed, anxious, distressed, guilty, angry, and physically diminished. When the fire dies out in a relationship because of a man's sexual dysfunction, he may not realize that his partner also has a personal involvement with the problem—even to the point of developing his or her own sexual disorder(s).

According to a recent study carried out at the University of Edinburgh, among all factors, sexual dysfunction was rated the number one cause of marital problems. Sex constitutes the flame that lights up marital life with its scintillating luster and bonds the couple together in love, complicity, and affection, and its loss may have a devastating effect on both people. They may elect to ignore the problem or to face it and find a solution. How can the sexually dysfunctional man and his partner best understand their situation and go about resolving it?

REACTIONS OF THE MAN TO HIS SEXUAL DYSFUNCTION

A popular joke reflects the not-so-funny frustration of a man having sexual difficulties: "What is the difference between anxiety and panic?" Answer: "Anxiety is the first time you cannot have it the second time—panic is the second time you cannot have it the first time."

A man with erectile or other sexual dysfunction may wallow in the pits of hell and may lose his self-esteem, self-confidence, and pride. He may experience painful frustration; a sense of the loss of his much-valued virility and manhood; and increased vulnerability to emotional, marital, familial, professional, and social difficulties. The radiant spring of his life may change to a cold, gloomy winter. He may shun any sex-related subject in normal conversation, and even with his physician, for fear of embarrassment. He may accuse his wife or partner of being the primary cause of his problem or deny its occurrence and refuse to discuss it or seek medical help. Within the relationship, the vital ingredients of intimacy, romanticism, love, and respect can gradually dwindle or be washed away by feelings of suspicion, blame, anger, repulsion, and even hatred. Physical and mental quality of life may be greatly reduced for the affected male and for the couple, subjecting them to significant emotional and psychological disturbances.

Fortunately, those feelings are not manifested by all men suffering from sexual dysfunction. Some of them may admit their problem and seek advice for any number of reasons. They may be motivated by a genuine desire to resume adequate sexual functioning, or they may be primarily worried about their physical health and only interested in ruling out any serious disease possibly underlying the dysfunction. They may seek professional help at the insistence of their partners, whether to please them, for reassurance, or for other psychological reasons. They may simply wish to regain their sense of manhood. But surprisingly, the majority of men with sexual dysfunction seem simply to accept their condition and refuse any medical help, with less than 12% of them attempting any safe, successful medical treatment for their distressing condition.

Contrary to false popular beliefs, sexual intercourse remains an important part of life for elderly people. About 30% to 70% of folks over 60 still engage in sexual relationships, with about 40% of men in their seventies having sex once a week (Braun M et al. 2000). According to several surveys by M. Perelman et al. (2005) of men aged 50–70, sex was rated by 13% as very important, by 29% as important, and by 41% as occasionally enjoyable; only 17% stated that they could live without it. Most of the men surveyed agreed that sexual dysfunction caused them and their partners great sadness and that it was important to assess their capabilities to perform sexually. Half reported that they would "do almost anything to cure their [erectile dysfunction]." Men in the United States and the United Kingdom were the most motivated to seek medical advice and find a cure (Perelman M et al. 2005).

In another study from the Netherlands on 1,481 men over the age of 18, the global prevalence of erectile dysfunction (ED) was 14.2%. Of those men, 67.3% were bothered by their condition, 68.7% either ignored it or accepted it as a natural phenomenon related to such things as their age, and 85.3%

wanted help. Unfortunately, only 10.4% of the afflicted men received any medical care for their condition (de Boer BJ et al. 2005). Nevertheless, these findings underscore the importance of sex at any age for men's well-being and quality of life.

Furthermore, several studies have demonstrated a positive correlation between successful sex and good general health, happiness, healthy relationships, intimacy, increased quality of life, decreased symptoms of depression, and positive self-image (Sadovsky R, Mulhall JP 2003). Physical and mental health, sexual intimacy, everyday interactions with women, sexual fantasy life, and men's perception of their masculinity are deeply affected by sexual disturbances, and sexually dysfunctional men have a higher incidence of anxiety and depression (Latini DM et al. 2002). ED's psychological impact may lead to reduced physical and emotional satisfaction, decreased general happiness, a decline in physical and mental health, and disturbed sexual and other personal relationships—all of which could be corrected with the resumption of normal sexual functioning (Seidman SN, Roose SP 2001).

It is important for sexual partners to be aware of the various psychological reactions that men with ED or other sexual dysfunctions may go through, so that they are better able to understand and sympathize. A man's reaction to his erectile failure is often devastation and humiliation. He may lose his confidence in his abilities and adequacy as a man. His self-esteem, ego, and self-worth may be crushed, and this may pave the way to depression, bringing with it additional stress and hostility toward himself and his partner. Beyond his sex life, his ED may impair not only his mental attitude, but also his professional and social relationships.

HOW DOES A MAN'S SEXUAL PROBLEMS AFFECT HIS PARTNER?

When suddenly confronted with a man's sexual problem, his partner's first reaction might be to ignore it, believing that it is only temporary and due to such causes as fatigue, illness, stress, alcohol, or perhaps an argument. If the problem persists, the partner starts to worry; everyone generally likes to have his or her world in order and may be inclined to search deeper for a reason for any dysfunction. "Is he having an affair? Doesn't he love me any more?" These thoughts are a common reaction. Partners of sexually dysfunctional men may become angry and resentful, feeling rejected and frustrated. It is not unusual for them to experience their own loss of self-respect and self-esteem and to question their own self-worth.

As the problem persists, partners often become increasingly concerned about its causes and possible consequences. They may attribute the dysfunction to an affair or a lack of desire or love on the man's part, or blame themselves. These ideas stir up further reactions of disappointment, insecurity, and distrust. Partners may conclude that they have failed in their relationship or marriage and wonder whether it will last. Tormented by these thoughts and feelings, they may behave as if in a state of defeat. They may decide to go back to ignoring it and hope for its spontaneous resolution. They may be too embarrassed to discuss it, or they may have tried to bring it up with the sufferer but to no avail. At this point, some people may become content with the situation, and even be relieved to give up sex.

Alternatively, partners of sexually dysfunctional men may start looking for information, sympathy, reassurance, understanding, and the best way to solve the problem. They may wonder about where to seek help, whom to trust, and whether it is possible to resolve the situation independently. They may talk about it with friends, clergymen, close relatives, or physicians; they may read about it or tune in to a TV program on the subject. Learning that the sexual dysfunction may be caused by a medical condition or disease can, unfortunately, increase their anxiety and agitation, potentially complicating the problem and further straining the relationship.

When people lack the correct information about a problem, they may feel that the problem is monstrous or incurable. Fear, hopelessness, and desperation may overcome rational thought and appropriate behaviors. Partners of sexually dysfunctional men may react to their mates in an unpredictable manner—perhaps avoiding sex, or demanding it persistently, or trying different ways to attract him—or they may decide to play an active role in seeking professional help. Some of them may develop their own sexual disturbances, which may improve following the successful treatment of their male partners.

POSITIVE WAYS FOR COUPLES TO DEAL WITH THE MAN'S SEXUAL DYSFUNCTION

One positive aspect of all the turmoil surrounding a man's sexual dysfunction may be a smart decision on his and his partner's part to seek professional help. This means that both people have acknowledged the problem and are motivated to solve it to save their relationship. Let me review some important facts as a starting place for seeking assistance and treatment.

First of all, they should both realize that for most men, erectile ability is synonymous to virility and manhood, and its loss may be one of the most devastating and humiliating experiences they may suffer. A few men with ED may even undergo surgical insertion of penile prostheses, without necessarily even using them for intercourse after surgery, simply to be satisfied that they are "men" again.

When a man has ED, his sexual partner is also affected by the dysfunction and may develop sexual problems as well. According to a study at Loyola

University's Sex Clinic, 52% of female partners of men with ED developed their own sexual problems after the onset of their partners' disorder (Renshaw DC 1981). The partner's reaction may be one of loneliness, isolation, doubt, rejection, and guilt. It is important for the couple to engage in cognitive restructuring to alleviate these negative emotions and solve the problem appropriately.

The partner should not feel guilty or totally responsible for the sufferer's sexual dysfunction. She or he should concentrate instead on being supportive and finding a solution, rather then being obsessed with the problem or trying to solve it alone. Both people must accept that no cure is possible until the man honestly acknowledges his problem and is willing to discuss it with his partner and seek medical help. His partner should feel compassion for his frustrations and should also realize that any lack of expressed emotions or manifestations of love, even his irritability and rejection of sexual advances, are probably results of his ED.

By being fully informed and enlightened about sexual dysfunctions, the partner can take an active role in seeking help and encouraging the afflicted man to seek medical advice early on. A sexual problem may be the first manifestation of a serious disease that should be diagnosed and treated promptly to prevent dangerous, or even fatal, consequences. In the meantime, the sufferer should keep in mind that his partner may still nurture a strong desire for him, and that it may be possible to have an orgasm and ejaculate without an erection. The couple should still engage in nonintercourse sexual activities that minimize any performance pressure and continue to manifest plenty of love, warmth, and respect toward each other.

Unfortunately, some people are totally unconcerned by their partners' sexual dysfunction and disinterested in participating in its management. Many may even prefer the situation as it is, for various reasons, including lack of sexual pleasure with their husbands, lack of interest in sex, satisfaction with an extramarital relationship, or refusal of all current artificial therapeutic methods that minimize their role in the sexual act. If either person in a relationship affected by ED resists assistance, it may be advisable for the other person to participate in a support group or seek the help of a sex therapist.

Clearly ED and other sexual dysfunctions have an impact on both individuals involved. Talking about the afflicted man's feelings can stir up some difficult emotions in his partner: sorrow for him, perhaps self-pity as well, or frustration, depression, anxiety, or failure as a lover. The couple must remember that the problem affects them both and that they may have similar feelings of inefficacy, sadness, and low self-esteem. These feelings, which are normal and to be expected under the circumstances, can be transient, disappearing following the dysfunction's successful treatment. There are, however, cases in which these emotional sequelae linger beyond the resolution of the sexual problem and may need to be addressed via self-help psychology or professional counseling.

Understanding the Problem and Its Causes

In many cases of ED, a man may feel aroused, excited, and ready for sex, but, when it comes to implementing his desire, his penis fails him. Evaluation and identification of any sexual dysfunction—ED, ejaculatory disorders, low libido, and others—is, of course, the first step on the road to successful treatment. As noted in chapter 5, ED may be due to various physical or psychological factors, or both.

Physical causes include aging (though ED is not an inevitable consequence of growing old); cardiovascular disease or ischemic heart disease; diabetes or other hormonal, vascular, or neurologic disease; hypertension and/or high cholesterol; lower urinary tract symptoms secondary to benign prostatic hyperplasia; chronic renal failure; pelvic injury (especially to the pelvic nerves); chronic alcoholism, drug abuse, or heavy smoking; obesity; and certain medications such as some of the antihypertensives, antidepressants, antipsychotics, female hormones, muscle-building steroids, and peptic ulcer drugs. ED may also occur following certain surgical procedures or result from chemotherapy or radiation therapy. (Physical causes of ED are detailed in chapter 7.)

The numerous psychological causes of ED include anxiety, stress, depression, Oedipal issues, fear, guilt, and various psychological inhibitions. Any of these can be activated by sexual excitement, which results in erectile difficulties because such psychogenic signals can inhibit the activation of the parasympathetic nerves and increase the activity of sympathetic nerves, leading to constriction of the penile arteries and therefore penile flaccidity. Marital discord, lack of communication, financial trouble, adultery, the practice of heterosexual sex by a homosexual man, physical repulsion, poor hygiene, and even rudeness may play major roles in ED's onset. Other psychological roots can be found in the ED sufferer's upbringing, experience of severe sanctions against sexual expression, erroneous beliefs about sex, and fear of failure and rejection by the sexual partner. A particular factor in many cases is the man's inability to abandon himself to a sexual experience; during sex, he may be obsessed with the quality of his performance or act as a spectator rather than an active participant. (Psychological factors are detailed in chapter 8.)

The next obvious question is, what can be done about it? Whether the ED is organic, psychogenic, or a combination of the two, most cases can be treated successfully, regardless of the man's age and underlying disease(s)—provided that he is willing and eager to be treated, is fit physically to engage in sex, and does not suffer from severe cardiovascular or other conditions that preclude engaging in sex.

Partners in Treatment

Physical conditions contributing to ED necessitate a thorough medical workup for diagnosis (chapter 9) and treatment (chapters 10 through 14). When ED is due to physical causes, it can be treated with oral drugs, vacuum devices, intracorporeal injections, intraurethral inserts, vascular surgery, or the insertion of a penile prosthesis. But it should be noted that in a substantial number of cases, behavioral changes such as smoking cessation, daily exercise, treating obesity, lowering serum cholesterol, curing alcohol and drug addiction, and substituting or changing medications by the treating specialist may restore the man's erectile ability without the need for any further therapy.

When ED is caused by psychological factors, treatment varies from behavioral and psychoanalytic therapy to sexual and marital therapy. Several psychological tactics to relieve performance anxiety; modify behavior; improve sexual communication between partners; acquire sexual skills; and eliminate taboos, misconceptions, and negative attitudes toward sex are employed (see chapter 14). Full cooperation of the couple is required for successful treatment.

A man's willingness to undergo treatment for a sexual problem should be seen as a special demonstration of his love, to which his partner should respond in the most loving and caring way. A couple's mutually positive and supportive attitude, based on complete understanding of the various aspects of sexual functioning and its disturbances and on a genuine desire to resume a fulfilling sex life, will affect the ultimate outcome. It is always preferable for both partners to discuss the preferred mode of treatment before its application to avoid any dissatisfaction or inhibition from its subsequent use and to gauge expectations against practicality.

Some partners of sexually dysfunctional men may feel uncomfortable with or even reject certain forms of therapy for ED, perhaps feeling that the erections created by these methods do not represent the God-given, natural erectile process based on a genuine physical and mental attraction. They may feel that they have lost their role in eliciting their partners' erections, depriving them of the pleasure of feeling desired and attractive. They may come to see the sex act under these circumstances as tainted and unnatural. Others worry about the possible medical side effects of the therapeutic methods on the man's health and well-being, or on their own. Some women, for instance, are concerned about the possibility of damaging the penile implant or being injured by the plastic ring used with the vacuum device.

Women who have never been truly interested in sex may abhor the idea of their partner recovering full potency, having more desire, and/or prolonging his erections. They may not be able to cope with his rejuvenated sexual capability, or they may worry (rightly or wrongly) that it will lead him to seek sexual pleasure with others. Some women seem quite satisfied with their partner's ED, perhaps because it enables them to avoid sex, instill feelings of guilt in their partner, control him physically and emotionally, or enjoy the role of a suffering victim.

There are certainly other factors for female dissatisfaction with their partners' renewed sexual vigor, such as financial/reproductive considerations, myths regarding the unimportance of sex in older age, or fear of betrayal. It is, however, very fortunate that many women are fully understanding, caring, and willing to participate actively in their partners' therapy and recovery and fully support the man's eagerness to regain his sexual ability so they can resume a happy, fulfilling sex life.

In conclusion, I must emphasize that optimal sexual functioning does not imply only a firm, erect penis, but must be viewed within a broader picture of shared love, intimacy, respect, physical and mental attraction, strong relationship dynamics, privacy, motivation, receptivity for sex, absence of performance anxiety or guilt or anger, and proper sexual communication. Any psychiatric, interrelational, emotional, marital, professional, and social disturbances must be effectively addressed to individualize treatment and optimize its outcome.

MEN'S REACTION TO ERECTILE DYSFUNCTION

Do you suspect that you might have erectile or other sexual dysfunction? You may be one of the 30 million American men suffering from ED. If so,

You may erroneously believe that is just the way life has rolled the dice for you.

You may have become resigned to your fate and have adapted yourself, possibly even with your sexual partner's approval, to a life without sex.

You may have heard that there is no cure for ED and that all the modes of treatment are just artificial means of improving your sexual functioning.

You may not like the idea of trying any treatments, despite their high efficacy and proven safety, perhaps because of personal reasons (such as not considering treatment worthwhile) or because of their cost.

You may have reacted to your sexual problem by avoiding sex entirely and replacing it with hobbies such as golf, painting, or reading, for your own, and even your partner's, satisfaction.

You may have avoided expressing affection to your partner, feeling that this might lead to an unsuccessful sexual encounter.

You may have fallen prey to the popular misconception that it is all in your head and that there is nothing physically wrong with you.

You may not be aware that almost every man with a sexual dysfunction, regardless of cause or age, can be helped to resume a fulfilling sex life, and that the majority of cases of ED can be successfully managed with appropriate therapy.

You may have accepted one or more of the common sexual fallacies and myths, for example, that you are too old for sex, that ED is inevitable with advancing age, or that sexual dysfunction is caused by past infidelity or excessive masturbation.

You may have lost self-confidence to such an extent that, if you are a single man, you
avoid dating and social activities that could lead to a sexual situation and failure.

You may believe there is a magic pill or other means of completely curing your dysfunction, or that it will soon be available, so you have decided to wait for it.

You may be too embarrassed to face your problem or to talk about it with your sexual
partner, your personal physician, or anyone else.

You may have been rebuffed by a doctor when you attempted to bring up the subject
of your sexual problems. Unfortunately, many doctors are too embarrassed to
discuss the topic or even to inquire about its occurrence with their patients.

You may consider yourself a failure in your relationship with your sexual partner.

You may have been misinformed regarding male sexual dysfunction—this misinfor-
mation is all too common. Not all medical professionals have any more knowledge and understanding of the subject than the average layperson.

Your partner's reaction to your dysfunction may have increased your worry and anxiety, adding to feelings of incompetence, loss of self-esteem and confidence, and
depression.

You may not have given much thought to the fact that male sexual dysfunction is not
just your problem but has an impact on your partner as well. It is erroneous, and
selfish, to believe that your sexual dysfunction only concerns you.

You may be satisfied with having orgasm without erection by using various sexually
stimulating techniques.

You may even like the way things are, despite the deep frustration, loss of self-esteem
and confidence, distress, bitterness, hostility, guilt, anger, disappointment, despair,
anxiety, and depression that it may be causing you and/or your partner.

Having an erectile or other sexual dysfunction, however, does not mean
that you cannot and should not continue to show love, warmth, and respect for
your partner—and receive it as well. To the extent that you are both willing,
you can continue to engage in nonintercourse activities. Your partner may still
have strong sexual desires and needs, despite your lack of erectile ability. Most
men can continue to have an orgasm and ejaculate without an erection.

If you are experiencing sexual difficulties, seek help from a medical expert,
who will be able to diagnose the problem correctly and recommend the best
treatment for you. Contrary to some misconceptions shared by some laypeople
and some nonexpert physicians, ED can be cured in many cases, sometimes
simply by the discontinuation of certain medications (or other drugs), smoking cessation, exercise, weight loss, male hormone supplementation, surgical
repair of a ruptured lumbar disk, or microsurgical arterial shunting for traumatic occlusion of the arteries providing blood to the penis.

Chapter Seven

PHYSICAL CAUSES OF ERECTILE DYSFUNCTION

The enjoyment of sex, although great/Is in later years said to abate/But how would I know?/I'm only seventy-eight.

Anonymous

To recognize erectile dysfunction (ED) and understand its causes, it is important to remember that penile erection is a continuous neurovascular phenomenon under psychological control and requires a proper hormonal milieu for its successful achievement. Recall these physiological mechanisms of erection, described previously: under sexual stimulation, impulses from the parasympathetic and nonadrenergic/noncholinergic (NANC) nerves cause the release of nitric oxide (NO, also possibly secreted from the penile vessels' endothelial cells). NO enters the smooth muscle cells inside the vessels in the corpora cavernosa, where it stimulates the enzyme guanylate cyclase to produce cyclic guanosine monophosphate. This activates the enzyme protein kinase G to phosphorylate (add a phosphate group) to certain proteins that are responsible for regulating the tone of the smooth muscles in the corporeal arteries and sinuses, thereby contributing to the relaxation of those vessels and the consequent inrush of blood to the penis.

By extension, you can see that any disease, injury, or disorder affecting the brain, nervous system, vascular system, endocrine system, smooth muscle of the corpora, tunica albuginea, neurotransmitters, or genitourinary system can lead to a man's inability to obtain or maintain a firm or rigid erection for enough time to ensure sexual gratification for himself or his partner. It may also lead to his disinterest in sexual activity. (Most men may experience some difficulty in achieving and maintaining an erection at some point in their lives; such transient episodes should not be considered a sign of ongoing ED (Lewis R et al. 2004, Lue TF 2004b, Shabsigh R et al. 2005a).

PATHOPHYSIOLOGY

The wide range of organic causal factors of ED may be categorized into four general types of conditions:

1. The inability to pump enough blood inside the penis, due to arterial disease, is the most common organic cause of ED, with an incidence of about 40%.
2. Neurologic conditions can prevent the penile nerves' normal secretion of the neurotransmitters that relax the penile arteries and sinuses or can decrease sensation in the penile nerves, thereby precluding activation of the erectile process. (Montorsi F et al. 2003)
3. Leakage of blood from abnormal penile veins during erection prevents the storage of blood inside the penis for a sufficient period. This leakage can be due to any pathology of the tunica, poor relaxation of the vascular sinuses, or fibrosis of the smooth muscle in the corpora.
4. Any medical condition that affects the penile arteriogenic system can lead to its failure to dilate and fill with a large volume of blood under high pressure.

Several medical conditions are clearly associated with an increased risk of ED. One report, for example, shows the following high prevalences: ED occurs in 52% of men with hypertension, 55% of men with urinary tract symptoms, 61% of men with ischemic heart disease, 64% of men with diabetes, 86% of men with peripheral vascular disease, and 90% of men with depression (Carson CC et al. 2006). This chapter details the various major risk factors associated with ED.

AGING

It is well accepted that ED's prevalence and severity increase with advancing age. Men over the age of 50 are usually afflicted by various organic conditions, including cardiovascular disease (CVD), diabetes, hypertension (high blood pressure), hypercholesterolemia (high cholesterol), and low testosterone; lower urinary tract symptoms (LUTS) secondary to benign prostatic hyperplasia (BPH); chronic neurologic conditions such as parkinsonism, stroke, and Alzheimer's; and psychological disorders such as depression and anxiety. Any of these, as well as the use of multiple medications, may contribute to ED. About 48% of men over 50 are affected by different degrees of ED due to physical, intrapsychic, and relational factors (Corona G et al. 2004)—but this does not mean that sexual dysfunction is an inevitable consequence of aging. In the majority of men over 50, sexual interest and desire remain strong.

A specific major risk factor for ED in men 50 and older is atherosclerosis of the pudendal and cavernosal arteries. This involves the formation of plaques in the arterial walls, gradually obstructing the lumen (the open space for blood flow). Atherosclerosis can be secondary to diabetes, hypertension, and hyper-cholesterolemia as well as to smoking. Atherosclerosis may lead to pathologi-cal changes such as penile smooth muscle degeneration and replacement by fibrous tissue, with reduced expandability of the corpora cavernosa, leading to venous leakage (Montorsi F et al. 2003).

Prostate problems are another specific risk factor in the aging male. Several recent studies confirmed a close association between sexual dysfunction—namely, ED, ejaculatory incompetence, hypoactive sexual desire, and painful ejaculation—and moderate or severe LUTS secondary to the BPH that com-monly occurs in over 50% of men after age 50. In some cases, treatment with certain alpha-blockers, Viagra, or Cialis has improved both the urinary and sexual symptoms. ED, ejaculatory problems, and LUTS may all stem from sympathetic nervous system overactivity, prostate infection or inflammation, vascular disorders in the penis and prostate, or a deficiency of NO. Typical prostate symptoms are pain in the pelvis, suprapubic area, perineum, ingui-nal area, scrotum, lower abdomen, and back as well as other BPH-associated symptoms such as burning on urination, frequency and/or urgency of urina-tion, and slow urine stream.

Normal age-related physiological changes are often falsely interpreted as sexual dysfunction, when they may actually require no more than full under-standing by the man and his partner and a readjustment in sexual techniques. Natural changes in a healthy man's sexual functioning with age include the following:

A progressive decline in free testosterone level, caused by a decreased testicular production of testosterone, which may affect erectile and orgasmic function and decrease libido.

A need for more genital stimulation to elicit erection, caused by a decreased sensitiv-ity of the penis to touch and vibration and an increased conduction time of the nerve impulses.

A need for more time to develop an erection, caused by a loss of elasticity in the penile arteries and sinuses and possibly by a decline in autonomic nervous system function.

A decrease in the hardness of the penis during erection, but with rigidity still ade-quate for penetration and successful intercourse, and no change in the circumfer-ential increase of the erect penis.

An increased time from excitation to ejaculation and a need to wait hours or even a few days before being able to develop a second erection.

A decline in the intensity of orgasm.

A decrease in the volume of ejaculated semen, caused mainly by atrophy of the pros-tate and seminal vesicular glands due to low serum testosterone (some older men may even stop ejaculating any semen at all, despite having good orgasms).

A reduction in the number, duration, and quality of spontaneous erections during sleep, perhaps due to a decrease in required total sleep time.

With the physical and mental slowing that usually accompanies aging, men can experience a loss of self-esteem, severe anxiety, depression, stress, and a sense of inadequacy. These feelings, when not appropriately counteracted by coping mechanisms, may lead to psychogenic sexual inadequacy. A lack of sexual interest on the part of their partners (perhaps suffering from sexual disturbances themselves) also contributes to some men's ED. In elderly men, relational problems, partner unavailability or unreceptiveness, and psychogenic disturbances such as depression, stress, or anxiety may play important causal roles in ED.

It is a misconception and a cruel myth that a man over the age of 60 cannot (or should not) function sexually. Older men need as much affection, love, understanding, tenderness, and privacy as younger men do, and perhaps more. Several studies have demonstrated that over 65% of men and women over the age of 65 are still interested in sex and are sexually active. They should be encouraged to express their sexual needs and to enjoy a fulfilling sex life without any feeling of shame or guilt. (When a sexual partner is not available, masturbation can be used to relieve sexual tensions.) It has been reported that the number of sexual encounters declines by about 75% between the ages of 30 and 65 but also that the majority of men over 60 report having regular sexual intercourse.

On the other hand, men over 60 certainly have a higher incidence of erectile failure than younger men. About 40% to 70% of men aged 40–70 complain of sexual dysfunction, with a marked decrease in frequency of sexual events after age 50. Causes of ED in this age group may include low free serum testosterone and vascular, hormonal, neurologic, psychological, and social factors. It is estimated that, despite reported sexual desire in more than 50% of males over the age of 80, less than 15% engage in sexual intercourse because of erectile failure.

A sexual and medical history and a physical examination are needed to elucidate the true nature of whatever sexual dysfunction a man may experience later in life, whether his major complaint is decreased libido, ejaculatory or orgasmic disturbance, or an erectile problem. Vascular, neurogenic, hormonal, and psychogenic factors must be assessed (and excluded) by specific testing. Therapy can then be tailored to the underlying cause of the dysfunction.

CARDIOVASCULAR CAUSES

Any severe narrowing, hardening, or clogging of the aorta, iliac vessels, and tributaries, or the penile arteries and sinuses, may result in sexual dysfunction. Vascular disease is the most common organic cause of ED, with a prevalence of about 40% of all organic factors.

About 17% of men with ED suffer from atherosclerosis, a clogging of the arteries with yellowish plaques containing cholesterol, lipoid (fatty) material, and lipophages (cells that absorb fat), which can lead to the partial or total obstruction of blood vessels. This common condition is usually associated with smoking, hyperlipidemia (elevated concentrations of any or all lipids in the blood, including cholesterol and triglycerides), obesity, and diabetes. The diminished blood flow in the penile arteries and sinuses prevents the engorgement and tumescence of the penis. It may also cause venous leakage because of poor compression of the venules against the tunica, secondary to contracted vascular sinuses.

Furthermore, a direct correlation has been found between CVD and ED (Montorsi F et al. 2006). The sexual problem may be the first sign of the presence of an occult (hidden) cardiac condition, such as ischemic heart disease, and may antedate its other clinical manifestations for months or years. This is why the penis is called the "body's barometer" of vascular integrity. The close correlation between ED and other vascular pathology has prompted some physicians to suggest a complete cardiovascular workup for any man suffering from ED, especially if he has risk factors such as smoking, diabetes, hypertension, obesity, and hyperlipedemia.

Patients with single-vessel ischemic heart disease have better erections than those with multiple-vessel obstruction. Furthermore, men with cavernous arterial insufficiency have a significantly higher risk of developing coronary arterial disease (CAD; Speel TG et al. 2003). Other atherosclerosis-associated factors, such as reduced endothelial NOS (nitric oxide synthase, an enzyme which converts L-arginine and oxygen to produce nitric oxide), increased levels of free radicals, and high concentration of homocysteine in the vascular plaques, may contribute to ED (Kendirci M et al. 2005). Strong recent evidence suggests that depletion of NOS from the nitrergic nerves (the NANC nerves in the penis that secrete NO) may also contribute to sexual dysfunction. Other CVDs, such as congestive heart failure and aortic aneurysm (formation of an abnormal sac in the aorta's wall), may be associated with ED.

A recent study analyzed the incidence of extragenital vascular disease in 457 patients with ED, based on echo Doppler ultrasound studies of penile arteries and carotid or lower-leg vessels suspected to contain atherosclerotic plaques. The researchers found isolated penile artery insufficiency in about 25% of the ED patients and combined penile, carotid, and lower-extremity atherosclerosis in 75% of the cases (Vicari E et al. 2005), again demonstrating a close relationship between vascular changes in the penile arteries and other arteries in the body.

In a recent Italian study, number of diseased coronary arteries, age, and diabetes were found to be independent factors in ED; ED, in turn, was associated with a fourfold risk of having CAD, as diagnosed by coronary angiography independently of other recognized risk factors. ED is frequently found in men with acute coronary syndromes and can be considered a sign of diffuse and/or coronary atherosclerosis (Montorsi F et al. 2006).

In another study, the most common vascular risk factor for the development of ED was smoking, followed by obesity and hypertension. The poorest blood flow and arterial insufficiency parameters were found in those men with ED who also had CAD (40% of the group), followed by those who also had diabetes (23.3%). Venous occlusive disease was observed in hypertensive patients (36.5%). The odds of having abnormal blood flow parameters increased with the number of vascular risk factors (Kendira M et al. 2006).

NEWSFLASH: ERECTILE DYSFUNCTION, CORONARY ARTERIAL DISEASE, AND CARDIOVASCULAR DISEASE

The association of erectile dysfunction (ED) with subsequent coronary arterial disease (CAD) in 9,457 men over 55 was reported by Thompson et al. (2006) at the American Urological Association's 2006 annual meeting. At the start of the study, ED was noted in 57% of the men. At five-year follow-up, 11% of the men with ED had experienced a cardiovascular disease (CVD) or cardiac event such as angina; myocardial infarction; high serum low-density lipoprotein, or LDL; cerebrovascular accident; or congestive heart failure. Therefore the hazard ratio (increased odds of acquiring a particular disease, expressed as a numeral above the normal value of 1) for CVD was 1.30 for the men with ED. The study's authors advocate prompt investigation and intervention for men with ED who also have risk factors for CAD or CVD.

As discussed earlier, a venous leak during erection means that blood that should normally remain trapped in the penis until detumescence (loss of erection) actually escapes at the beginning of an erection or soon after its development, resulting in ED. This may be caused by leakage of blood through congenitally abnormally large veins; dysfunction or injury of cavernous smooth muscle secondary to trauma, diabetes, or atherosclerosis; or tunica albuginea weakening due to aging or Peyronie's disease. Other neurogenic and psychogenic disorders that cause inadequate neurotransmitter release may also contribute to venous leakage, as can smoking, hypertension, high cholesterol, or an intrinsic pathology affecting the smooth muscles of the corpora. Venous leakage may be considered one of the major causes of ED, with an incidence of about 65% among men with ED.

A substantial number of men complain of unsustained erections; although they may develop a good erection, they lose it quite rapidly, often too soon for intercourse to be successful. Some of these men have a venous leak. This is in contrast to men whose ED is caused by insufficient arterial blood inflow. These men usually take a longer time to develop erections, and then, if they do achieve erections at all, they lose them more slowly. A combination of venous leakage and arterial disease is suspected in men who develop erections slowly and lose them rapidly.

To summarize, vasculogenic factors are the most common cause of organic ED. These include hardening or occlusion of the extrapenile arteries or the intrapenile vessels, hypertension, cholesterol (high levels of low-density lipoprotein, or LDL, or low levels of high-density lipoprotein, or HDL), or diabetes as well as pelvic trauma, surgery, or radiation therapy. Impaired erectile hemodynamics are reported in men with myocardial infarction (MI), coronary bypass surgery, peripheral vascular disease, cerebrovascular accident (CVA), and hypertension. The incidence of ED is about 60% in cases of MI and coronary bypass and about 10% in cases of untreated hypertension. The combination of risk factors such as diabetes, vascular diseases, hypertension, and smoking significantly increases the incidence of ED. Furthermore, as mentioned, the penis may serve as the main barometer of vascular endothelial anomalies in the rest of the body, and the occurrence of ED may herald the future development of CVD.

DIABETES MELLITUS

Some 30% to 75% of men with diabetes complain of ED, and conversely, statistics show that about one out of four men with ED has diabetes; in fact, a finding of ED may even lead to the initial discovery of a man's diabetes. In one study, ED was the first sign of diabetes in 12% of the study group, and 50% of the diabetics developed ED within 10 years of their diabetes diagnosis (Kaiser FE, Korenman SG 1988; Israilov S et al. 2005; De Berardis 2007).

Sexual dysfunction in diabetics has been found to be age-dependent, with ED affecting 15% of those aged 30–34, versus about 55% of 60-year-old diabetics (Whitehead ED, Kyde BJ 1990, De Berardis G et al. 2007). Type 2 diabetes, which usually occurs in older people and is due to insulin resistance, is associated with a higher incidence of ED than the hereditary type 1. A recent study covering 401 men with ED followed for a period from nine years, from 1987–1989 to 1995–1998, up to 15 years (2002–2004), with no treatment, in the Massachusetts Longitudinal Aging Study revealed some interesting and unexpected findings. While about 33% of men with minimal or moderate ED exhibited ED progression, about 32%, 14%, and 31% of men with minimal, moderate, and complete ED, respectively, recovered full sexual potency. Weight loss, cessation of smoking, and improvement of overall health were the most important factors involved in the remission of ED and/or delaying its progression (Travison TG et al. 2007).

Diabetes-associated ED may be multifactorial, with both organic and psychogenic causes. Among the most important organic factors in these cases are the following:

Vascular disease with atherosclerosis that may be associated with diabetes; such a condition could lead to the obstruction or narrowing of the penile arteries or to a venous leak.

A recent experimental study revealed that impairment of NOS, the principal enzyme responsible for the synthesis of NO in the endothelial cells in the penile vessels, may represent a major cause of diabetic sexual dysfunction.

Other important factors in diabetes-associated ED are neuropathies, which means that the nerves of the penis and their secretion of neurotransmitters may be adversely affected by the disease.

Some sexually dysfunctional diabetic men may suffer primarily from a deficiency of testosterone or from major psychogenic disturbances. A recent study demonstrated a strong link between ED, sensory neuropathy, and decreased sexual desire independent of age in some diabetics with ED. This suggests that psychogenic factors may have marked influence in cases of diabetic ED (Nakanishi S et al. 2004).

Recent electron microscope studies in diabetic men with ED revealed pathologic changes in the nerves and smooth muscles of the cavernous tissue and penile arteries. Impaired smooth muscle relaxation in the corpora cavernosa was demonstrated in cases of ED by researchers at Boston University Medical Center. In addition, recent studies indicate that diabetes and high cholesterol may prevent full relaxation of the trabecular smooth muscle in the penile vascular sinuses, with clogging of small intrapenile arteries in the cavernous tissue, which may lead to ED.

Additional causes of ED in men with diabetes include blood hypercoagulability, secretion of vasoconstrictive substances, and replacement of smooth muscle by collagen in the corpora. Recent studies have discovered new etiologic factors that may play a major role in the sexual impairment of diabetic patients, including endothelial dysfunction, oxidative stress, neuropathy, and structural changes (Kendirci M et al. 2005).

In diabetics, increased activity of the RhoA/Rho-kinase pathway, which regulates NOS expression from the endothelial cells and also functions in the corpora cavernosa, may inhibit NO production. Overproduction of advanced glycation end-product in diabetics may also decrease the production of NO. Overproduction of reactive oxygen radicals, which can cause neurovascular deficits, and overaction of the protein kinase C pathway (involving an enzyme of the transferase class that helps produce enzymes and proteins by phosphorylation inside the cells) have also been suggested as possible causes of diabetic ED (Kendirci M et al. 2005).

Other endocrine diseases that may contribute to ED include hypogonadism, hypo- and hyperthyroidism, adrenal disorders, and hyperprolactinemia (see the following section on endocrine and hormone factors).

THE METABOLIC SYNDROME AND ERECTILE DYSFUNCTION

The metabolic syndrome was defined by a National Institutes of Health expert panel in 2001 and is characterized by the following clinical findings:

Waist circumference greater than 40 inches or 100 centimeters
Systolic blood pressure over 130 millimeters of mercury (mmHg; generated pressure that pushes a column of mercury up a tube from 0 to 200 mm high) and diastolic blood pressure over 85 mmHg; or the use of antihypertensive medications
HDL cholesterol less than 40 milligrams per deciliter; or the use of lipid-lowering medications
Self-reported diabetes
Triglycerides of more than 150 milligrams per deciliter

Metabolic syndrome has been demonstrated to be a precursor of cardiovascular disease (CVD), and it was found in 43% of the erectile dysfunction (ED) population, as opposed to about 24% of a matched population with an increased incidence of insulin resistance. Its early detection in younger men with ED but with no other clinical symptoms may reduce their risk of future endothelial dysfunction and CVD (Bansal TC et al. 2005). A recent study confirmed these findings and demonstrated that ED was predictive of the occurrence of the metabolic syndrome in men with a body mass index (BMI) of less than 25. This important finding emphasizes that ED could provide an early warning sign and the opportunity for early therapeutic intervention for aging men with ED who are considered, due to their low BMI, to be at higher risk of developing metabolic syndrome and subsequent CVD (Kupelian V et al. 2006a).

NEUROGENIC FACTORS

Neurologic conditions are causal factors in about 10% to 20% of ED cases. Various diseases and disorders may affect the brain's sex centers or other parts of the nervous system such as the hypothalamus, pituitary gland, spinal cord, and peripheral nerves supplying the penis, all of which play important roles in sexual development and function (see chapters 3–4). Brain lesions, for example, may disturb the secretion of vital neurotransmitters, such as dopamine and oxytocin, and inhibit the transmission of neural impulses from the sex centers to the penile nerves via the spinal cord. Causes of such lesions include stroke, Alzheimer's disease, tumor, epilepsy, CVA, infection, parkinsonism, multiple sclerosis (MS), and trauma.

Spinal cord lesions caused by conditions such as injury, tumors, infections, MS, diabetic neuropathy, herniated disk, and neurosyphilis may be associated with loss of psychogenic and possibly reflexogenic erections as well as absence of sexual pleasure, orgasm, and ejaculation. These problems are due to disturbed transmission of sensory impulses from the penis to the brain and motor stimuli from the brain to the penis. The severity of the dysfunction depends on the level and extent of the lesion, particularly in relation to the secondary sex center in the sacral spine. Any pathology involving the sacral sex center leads to the absence of both reflexogenic and psychogenic erections. Trauma to the pelvic or penile nerves, by disrupting passage of neural impulses to and from the penis, can cause sensation loss and ED.

In cases of spinal cord injury, it has been reported that about 70% of paraplegics or quadriplegics are sexually active and that about 70% of them practice alternate forms of sexual expression such as oral or genital stimulation. One study found that reflexogenic erections were present in about 95% of patients with spinal injuries above the sacral vertebrae, and that psychogenic erections were maintained in about 25% of patients with partial sacral injuries. Although erectile ability was preserved in about 90% of those patients with incomplete lesions, those erections were generally unpredictable and brief, with poor ejaculation, precluding normal sexual functioning.

HYPERTENSION

Several recent epidemiologic studies confirmed the correlation of hypertension and ED. In the past, it was estimated that about 8% to 10% of patients with untreated hypertension suffered from ED when first diagnosed with high blood pressure. More recent studies, however, have reported much higher prevalences, ranging from 26% to 41% (Rosen RC et al. 2004; Seftel AD et al. 2004). Hypertension may damage the NO-secreting vascular endothelium of the penile arteries or alter the composition of the tissue in the corpora cavernosa, leading to increased size and proliferation of the smooth muscles, increased inelastic collagen and fibrosis, and hyperactivation of the sympathetic nervous system. This may impair the ability of the penile vessels to relax and dilate to accommodate the high volume of blood necessary for erection.

Furthermore, a low level of serum testosterone, which is observed in some young hypertensive males, may alter the secretion of NO in the penile tissue, impair the responsiveness of the tissue to its action, or contribute to sexual dysfunction through the anxiety and fear it generates in the afflicted person. As an unfortunate side effect of treatment, some antihypertensive drugs, such as diuretics and certain beta-blockers, can decrease libido and exacerbate sexual dysfunction. This occurs when the drug causes a constriction of the penile arteries or when it has an antiandrogenic effect, affecting sexual desire and the ability to develop firm erections.

MEDICATIONS, DRUGS, AND ALCOHOL

Medications may represent ED's most common etiology, with an incidence of about 25%. The general categories of these drugs include the following:

- Antihypertensives
- Antiarrhythmics
- Antidepressants
- Antipsychotics
- Cholesterol-lowering drugs
- Anabolic steroids
- Anticonvulsants
- Chemotherapeutics
- Tranquilizers
- Diuretics (for water elimination)
- Cardiac drugs (such as digoxin)
- Anticholinergics (nerve impulse blockers)
- Peptic ulcer drugs (such as cimetidine)
- Antiandrogens (such as estrogens)
- Antidepressants
- Narcotics
- Some barbiturates and antihistamines

Several prescription medications adversely affect male potency, with some resulting in decreased sex drive and/or loss of erectile ability. The most common are antihypertensive drugs such as beta-blockers, diuretics, calcium channel blockers, and those acting centrally on the brain; some sedatives; GnRH (Gonadotropin releasing hormone) agonists used to treat advanced prostate cancer; 5-alpha reductase (Proscar or Avodart) for BPH treatment; and female hormones and antiandrogens. Among other medications associated with ED are H2 antagonists used for peptic ulcer, selective serotonin reuptake inhibitors and some other antidepressants, amphetamines, antiepileptics, and antipsychotics (Lobo JR, Nehra A 2005).

Certain over-the-counter drugs—for example, chronic use of vasoconstricting nasal decongestants—have been implicated in the development of sexual dysfunction. Use of illicit drugs (marijuana, cocaine, etc.) can cause ED as well. Small amounts of cocaine may produce sustained erections and delayed ejaculation, but chronic use of cocaine and/or opiates may lead to sexual dysfunction.

As for alcohol, minimal or moderate consumption may increase sexual enjoyment in about 45% of men and about 70% of women. Sexual arousal with alcohol consumption is usually affected by the individual's beliefs regarding alcohol's effect. However, chronic alcoholism, or even simply drinking large quantities of alcohol, may lead to ED, with decreased serum testosterone and increased female hormones. It may block the release of the pituitary and testicular hormones and affect the metabolism of the female hormone estrogen (in the form of estradiol) in the liver.

ENDOCRINE AND HORMONE FACTORS

As noted earlier, testosterone influences the development of the male's reproductive system and secondary sexual characteristics. It is needed, especially in its free, or bioavailable, form in the serum, by most males for sexual arousal and proper functioning of the sex organs. It also regulates the secretion of neurotransmitters from the sex centers in the brain and spinal cord and possibly the secretion of NO in the corpora (see chapter 16). Testosterone's involvement in erection and ED, however, is still a subject of controversy.

Experimental and clinical data show that an appropriate hormonal milieu (primarily testosterone) plays an active role in maintaining normal sexual functioning. Recent clinical studies measuring total testosterone levels demonstrate that about 5% of men complaining of ED may have low hormonal levels, while about 18% may have low levels of free testosterone (Martinez-Jabaloyas JM et al. 2006). Although testosterone is thought to facilitate erection by dilating the penile arterioles and vascular sinuses, its effect on the production of ED is still controversial (Mikhail N 2006). Elevated serum prolactin, a pituitary hormone, may cause almost 6% of ED cases and is usually associated with low testosterone. Hyper- or hyposecretion of thyroid hormones may cause sexual dysfunction as well.

The Massachusetts Male Aging Study (MMAS) assessed the impact of sex hormones on ED in 1,519 men, aged 40–70, at baseline. There was no association between total testosterone, bioavailable testosterone, and serum hormone-binding globulin (SHBG) with ED. Only increased levels of luteinizing hormone were associated with increased risk of ED, which may indicate a relationship between ED and testicular function independent of testosterone levels (Kupelian V et al. 2006b).

In certain cases, however, the major effect of decreased serum testosterone is reduced sex drive. Men who have everything intact but who have a decreased free testosterone level often get a sexual boost from a resupply of the hormone. Some older men with low serum testosterone and ED, however, may not respond to intramuscular testosterone injection. This is because most of the injected hormone binds to blood proteins such as SHBG, decreasing the free portion that can act on the tissues or causing a rapid increase in serum testosterone within 72 hours that gradually decreases over the next two to three weeks. Nowadays, optimal replacement that normalizes serum testosterone within 24 to 72 hours is achieved with patches, gel, mucoadhesive tablets, and some oral tablets.

Testosterone injections sometimes restore erectile ability in eunuchs, or in males who lost their testicles before puberty (before their bodies had manufactured testosterone for any great length of time) as well as in castrated men who lost their testicles postpuberty (after a much longer period of testosterone production). Although some castrated men may occasionally obtain and maintain adequate erections without supplemental testosterone, most do not.

As another important part of a healthful hormonal milieu, thyroid hormones can also affect sexual function and dysfunction. Excessive production of these hormones by thyroid gland overactivity (hyperthyroidism), or deficiency of these hormones due to thyroid gland underactivity (hypothyroidism), can lead to ED, loss of sexual desire, and ejaculatory disturbances.

SURGERY

In both male and female patients, surgery on the pelvis, rectum, or internal genitalia contribute to postoperative sexual dysfunction at incidences ranging from 8% to about 32%, depending on the type of surgery. Bilateral orchiectomy (removal of the testicles) for the treatment of advanced prostate cancer may cause ED by lowering testosterone to castrated levels. The nerves and blood vessels that contribute to the erectile process may be severed or injured in other surgical procedures such as retroperitoneal (beneath and behind the abdominal cavity) operations for abdominal aneurysm (an abnormal bulge in an arterial wall), aortoiliac bypass, or spinal cord surgery; radical prostatectomy (total removal of a cancerous prostate; used to treat early-stage prostate cancer, when the malignancy is usually confined to the prostate); simple prostatectomy for BPH; external sphincterotomy (surgical cutting of a sphincter muscle) for neurogenic bladder (secondary to spinal cord injury, stroke, or tumor); or radical surgery for bladder or rectal cancer.

In the particular case of radical prostatectomy, the incidence of postoperative ED varies from 20% to 100%, depending on the patient's age and presurgical erectile capabilities, the surgical preservation of the nerves that supply the penis, and the surgeon's experience. Furthermore, some patients may develop postoperative urinary incontinence during orgasm, which may cause them embarrassment and may make them shun any sexual encounter.

Other factors that may influence the return of normal erections after radical prostatectomy include use of phosphodiesterase drugs such as Viagra, Cialis, or Levitra, use of prostaglandin E1 injections or intraurethral inserts, or a combination of these medications, starting about four weeks after surgery; adequate sexual desire and interest in sex on the part of the patient; availability and willingness on the part of his sexual partner to engage in intercourse; and lack of anxiety, depression, or other psychogenic disturbances. At follow-up with patients 24 and 48 months after bilateral nerve-sparing surgery, erectile recovery ranged from about 32% to 80% (with or without pharmacological therapy).

PHYSICAL TRAUMA

Trauma to the pelvic or penile nerves from a vehicle accident, fall, gunshot wound, or pelvic fracture with bladder or urethral rupture may contribute to the development of ED. Spinal and brain injuries are discussed earlier in this chapter. A disruption of blood flow in the penile arteries can also result from an injury in adolescence such as a forceful crash of the crotch against the crossbar of a bicycle.

OBESITY, HYPERLIPIDEMIA, AND SMOKING

The bad news is that obesity associated with overeating, lack of exercise, a sedentary lifestyle, gluttony, and smoking may contribute to ED. The good news is that in about 30% of these cases, regular exercise, a balanced diet, cessation of smoking, and loss of weight may lead to recovery of sexual function without the need for any therapy.

While 26% of patients with ED have elevated serum cholesterol levels, this figure increases to about 40% to 80% if they also suffer from hypertension (Seftel AD et al. 2004). The exact mechanism for the loss of normal sexual functioning due to high levels of serum cholesterol is still unknown. Several theories, based on experimental studies in rats and rabbits, attribute their relationship to poor endothelium-dependent relaxation of the vascular bed; accumulation of the "bad" cholesterol (LDL) in plaques, clogging the penile arteries; fewer nerves or endothelial cells; and higher concentration of smooth muscle cells (Gholami SS et al. 2003). Other factors include neurologic and vascular changes, with atrophy and decreased number and size of axons (the projection by neurons emit impulses), cavernosal smooth cell degeneration, and loss of vascular endothelial growth factor (Kendirci M et al. 2005).

As for smoking, several studies have reported direct correlation between the number of cigarettes per day and the duration of smoking with ED's development and severity, even in the absence of other risk factors. Contributors to the sexual problem include deficient endothelium-dependent smooth muscle relaxation of the penile vasculature, narrowing of the pudendal arteries, and poor rigidity during nocturnal erections. Among other factors are impaired autonomic function, endothelial damage, vasospasm of the penile arteries, decreased concentrations of NOS and NO, and increased toxic free radicals and aromatic compounds, which may cause poor arterial blood flow or lead to venous leakage in the penis.

LOWER URINARY TRACT SYMPTOMS

Benign (noncancerous) enlargement of the prostate gland may actively or passively compress the urethra (urinary channel). LUTS of urinary frequency, urgency, slow stream, hesitancy, incomplete bladder emptying, straining, post-voiding dribbling, and sometimes incontinence occur in about 40% to 50% of men over 50 who have BPH. Those symptoms may be quite annoying and affect quality of life.

Recent studies correlated LUTS (according to their degree of severity) with ED, ejaculatory incompetence, and painful ejaculations. In a study surveying 12,815 men aged 50 to 80, called the Multinational Survey of the Aging Male and conducted in the United States and six European countries, the severity of the urinary symptoms constituted a major risk factor for the development of erectile and ejaculatory disturbances, irrespective of age and other risk factors (Rosen R et al. 2003). Several as yet unconfirmed theories attribute this correlation between urinary and sexual symptoms to hyperactivity of the sympathetic nervous system in the prostate and penis, resulting in excessive contraction of the prostatic smooth muscles and penile arteries; to lack of NO in both organs; or to atherosclerotic changes in the blood vessels, with a significant decrease in penile blood flow.

Recently, much emphasis has been placed on the Rho-kinase role in both ED and LUTS secondary to BPH. RhoA is a small guanosine triphosphate protein that regulates several cellular processes, including smooth muscle contraction. Morphological changes in the prostate, penis, and bladder in patients with ED or LUTS share a common mechanism, namely, the up-regulation of Rho-kinase activity in the urinary and genital tract. This up-regulation may lead to increased sensitivity to calcium and an elevated response to contractile transmitters and mediators.

As with hypertension, some medications used to treat urinary symptoms may affect sexual function. The 5-alpha reductases, such as Proscar (finasteride) and Avodart (dutasteride), may decrease sexual desire, affect sexual potency, and inhibit ejaculation. Alpha-blockers, particularly Flomax (tamsulosin), may produce ejaculatory disturbances in up to 30% of cases. This negative effect is believed to be due to the drug's inhibitory influence on the seminal vesicles and the vas deferens or to its central actions in the brain. On the other hand, uroselective alpha-blockers, such as Flomax and Uro-Xatral (alfuzocin), as well as phosphodiesterase type 5 inhibitors (see chapter 10) may improve both the urinary and sexual symptoms. However, as per U.S. Food and Drug Administration warnings, Viagra doses above 25 milligrams should not be taken within four hours of taking an alpha-blocker. Clinical studies have confirmed the safety of combining Cialis and Flomax, or Cialis and Uro-Xatral, for the simultaneous treatment of LUTS and ED, with no serious side effects.

PEYRONIE'S DISEASE

First described by French physician, Francois de la Peyronie, in 1743, this condition is characterized by a plaque or a patch of scar tissue that forms on the tunica albuginea and penetrates into the cavernous tissue. This plaque, depending on its location, may cause penile curvature (usually dorsal, possibly other directions) or sometimes an hourglass appearance due to indentation in the middle of the shaft, with possible narrowing from the indentation toward the glans penis. This deformity may lead to vascular anomalies, which may result in ED. If untreated for a long time, about 40% of Peyronie's disease cases progress, about 47% do not change, and about 13% spontaneously regress (Gelbard MK et al. 1990).

Peyronie's disease afflicts about 0.4% to 16% of men worldwide. In one study of 4,432 middle-aged German men, its incidence was about 3.2% (Sommer F et al. 2002). Despite extensive study, its etiology is still unknown, but there are several theories. One is genetic, based on the association of Peyronie's disease with a genetic condition called Dupuytren's contracture of the hands as well as with the presence of certain genes called HLA-B27 subtypes. Other theories include an autoimmune reaction forming antielastin antibodies against the body's own tissue, abnormal wound healing due to a genetic predisposition, and injury resulting in a plaque of collagen (the protein in the white fibers of connective tissue) (Pryor J et al. 2004).

Currently the most accepted theory of the etiology of Peyronie's disease is that repeated physical trauma during intercourse leads to bleeding, deposition of fibrin (a blood substance involved in the clotting process), inflammation in the tunica or beneath it at the septum dividing the corpora cavernosa, and overproduction of cytokines by inflammatory cells such as T lymphocytes. Cytokines are nonantibody proteins, such as platelet-derived growth factor and transforming growth factor, that contribute to an immune response by attracting other inflammatory cells, such as neutrophils, macrophages, and fibroblasts, to the site of injury. This inflammation results in overproduction of collagen and may inhibit the enzyme collagenase, which normally breaks it down. Other contributors to collagen overproduction and abnormal tissue remodeling during healing may be genetic anomalies, increased oxidative stress caused by overproduction of oxygen free radicals and possibly the enzymes (NOS isoforms) responsible for the production of NO, and obstruction of the draining vessels (Montorsi F 2005). Peyronie's disease is also associated with other risk factors such as hypertension, diabetes, dyslipidemia, smoking, and obesity.

Diagnosis and Treatment of Peyronie's Disease

Diagnosis of Peyronie's disease is based on symptoms of penile angulation, pain, and possible ED and on a past medical history of trauma to the penis or other medical conditions such as Dupuytren's contracture. Physical examination focuses on palpation (identification by touch) of the plaque in the tunica albuginea and possibly the estimation of its size and location with color Doppler ultrasonography, which can also confirm the vascular cause of the sexual dysfunction, if present. Demonstration of the degree of penile curvature during erection by a photograph or videotape taken at home, or by observation after intrapenile injection of a vasodilator in the doctor's office, may be very helpful in deciding on future management.

Management of Peyronie's disease depends on several factors: duration, degree of deformity, presence of pain or ED, and stage of disease. No surgical treatment is advisable before at least 12 months from onset, with the stabilization of the disease for at least 3 months. Clinical manifestations of the early stage include a palpable extended plaque with pain and penile deformity during erection. Manifestations of the late stage are a harder and more localized plaque (sometimes associated with calcification), stable penile deformity, and possible ED in about 30% of these cases (Ralph DJ, Minhas S 2004).

In a case of minimal deformity with no pain or discomfort, no treatment is indicated; the patient is simply reassured and receives periodic follow-up. In a case of pain, marked curvature, and possible ED, conservative management with oral medications, locally applied electroshock wave lithotripsy (ESWL, more commonly employed to disintegrate kidney or urinary stones), or intralesional injections may be attempted, although they are usually associated with varying degrees of success.

Several medications, such as colchicine, vitamin E, potassium aminobenzoate, tamoxifen, acetyl-L-arginine, steroids, antihistamines, and others, alone or in combination, have been tried with varying success rates, but to no definitive benefit, except occasional moderate improvement of pain and curvature, or the prevention of progression in the early stages of the disease. Injection of verapamil (a cardiac drug used for the treatment of angina and some arrhythmias) or interferon alpha-2 B (a family of glycoproteins with antiviral properties, used in the immunologic treatment of some cancers) in the plaque every 2 weeks for 12 weeks or more has yielded mixed results. One study reported decreased penile curvature in about 60%, increased penile girth in about 83%, and improved sexual function in 71% (Levine LA, Estrada CR 2002); another reported no apparent benefit compared to placebo (Greenfield JM et al. 2006). Combined verapamil injection and oral propionyl-L-carnitine was more effective than either treatment alone (Cavallini G et al. 2002).

Recently, experimental injection of subtypes of the enzyme collagenase into the plaque yielded preliminary good results and may become the future treatment of choice. Using ESWL on the plaques resulted in marked improvement in about 50% of cases, with patient satisfaction of 64% in one study (Manikandan R et al. 2002), but these findings were not universally corroborated by other authors, so this method remains experimental until its efficacy is further confirmed by well-controlled studies.

In the late stage with duration over 12 months, penile deformity severe enough to preclude penetration, and failure of all conservative treatments, surgical intervention may be indicated, if accepted by the patient after an explanation of all the benefits and risks. The major reconstructive surgical interventions, provided the disease is stable for at least three months, include plication procedures, plaque incision and grafting, incisional corporoplasty, and the insertion of penile prostheses with or without modeling. The choice of the surgical procedure depends on the nature of the deformity, the degree of curvature, the stability of the disease, the magnitude of the penile deformity, the length of the erect penis, and erectile function. Plication procedures are reserved for patients with generous length, simple curvature, and normal erection or erectile dysfunction responsive to pharmacotherapy. They are simple to perform, with good cosmetic results, preservation of preoperative rigidity, and a high patient satisfaction of 45% to 100%. Their major disadvantage is penile length loss, from 0.5 centimeters to 4 centimeters in 46% to 100% of cases, and the recurrence of the angulation in 20% to 45% of cases.

Plaque incision and grafting is reserved for cases with short penile length; severe and complex deformities, such as low glass appearance; and normal sexual functioning. Its advantages include penile length preservation in 60% to 80% of the cases and high patient satisfaction of 80% to 90%. Its disadvantages include a postoperative erectile dysfunction rate of 5% to 20% and penile sensory loss. Insertion of penile prostheses with possible modeling of the penis is indicated in the presence of ED unresponsive to pharmacotherapy, with an excellent success rate and high patient satisfaction in 80% to 100% of cases.

In summary, in the absence of ED and the presence of penile curvature of less than 60 degrees, with difficulty in penetration, provided the length of the penis is adequate, plication (excision of wedge-shaped pieces of the tunica from the convex side of the penis at the site of maximal curvature, with transverse resuturing of the defects in the tunica) yields good results in the majority of cases. If the curvature is over 60 degrees and/or the penis is small, making an incision in the plaque and grafting with various natural or synthetic materials (the grafting material may consist of veins, pericardium, tunica albuginea, collagen fleece, dermis, temporalis fascia lata, dura mater, bovine or porcine small intestine submucosa (PCIS). Moreover, a new study demonstrated the presence of nonpalpable scarring of the penile septum, considered an atypical form of Peyronie's disease, as visualized by duplex Doppler ultrasonography in 20 of 341 patients with unexplained ED (Bella AJ et al. 2006).

MISCELLANEOUS ORGANIC CAUSES

About 20% to 50% of patients treated for prostate cancer with external radiation or brachytherapy (the implantation of radioisotope seeds) subsequently develop ED. Other organic causes include arteriosclerosis (hardening of the arteries), chronic renal failure, liver failure, external or internal radiation therapy for rectal cancer, urethral rupture, and chronic obstructive lung disease. Bicycling regularly for extended periods of time may compress the internal pudendal artery against the symphysis pubis, causing hypoxia (poor oxygenation) of the penile tissue—especially if the rider leans forward—and may be associated with ED (Gemery JM et al. 2006).

Type 1 diabetes; testicular torsion (twisting) with necrosis (tissue death) during childhood; and chromosomal abnormalities such as XXY, XX, or XO chromosomal combinations in boys, instead of the normal XY, could also cause testicular deficiency, which may lead to ED and/or loss of sexual desire (see chapter 16).

Chapter Eight

PSYCHOLOGICAL CAUSES OF ERECTILE DYSFUNCTION

To fear love is to fear life, and those who fear life are already three parts dead.

Bertrand Russell

The pioneering work of Masters and Johnson in the 1970s shed significant new light on the possible causes of sexual dysfunction. Their publications emphasized the influence of religious orthodoxy, fear of failure, homosexuality, and maternal influence as contributors to erectile dysfunction (ED). Subsequent theories considered additional psychological factors such as the man's "thinking" about sex, negative self-image and expectations, the partner's needs and preferences, and the influence of marital conflict on sexual function.

Recent studies have stressed the importance of not only anxiety, but also various physical conditions as major causal factors in ED. Although about two-thirds of the causes of ED are organic, psychogenic issues are still a critical part of male sexual dysfunction, and experts have not completely forgotten them. Psychosocial, lifestyle, demographic, marital, developmental, religious, and pharmacological factors may play a major contributory role in ED's initiation or persistence, whether alone or, in a substantial number of cases, as a response to the sexual dysfunction. Emotional reactions to sexual dysfunction may be severe and should be addressed seriously in both the diagnosis and management of this devastating condition.

PSYCHOGENIC RISK FACTORS

Erectile failure may occur at any time during a man's development. He may acquire a poor self-image, low self-esteem, diminished sense of confidence, or desire to engage in perverted sexual practices. He may be overwhelmed by a domineering parental figure or influenced by religious fanaticism. A single episode of failure to perform may lead to a repetitive cycle of fear and failure, ultimately resulting in sexual dysfunction. Depression, anxiety, guilt, stress, worry, and relationship disturbances can affect sexual desire and may lead to ED. Additionally, psychogenic ED may be triggered by drug and alcohol abuse, or even (more rarely) by guilt and despair resulting from a vasectomy or by sexual abuse during childhood.

Prominent psychologist J. LoPicollo (1991) groups psychogenic issues that could affect male sexual functioning into two overall categories. In the first, he lists factors related to a man's personality, attitude, expectations, interest in sex, implicit or explicit demands for sex, attentional focus on erotic cues, sexual arousal, character, upbringing, psyche, and sexual behavior. Men having trouble with these factors include, for example, obsessive-compulsive individuals who have difficulty showing emotions during sex, those who find bodily secretions unpleasant, depressed men, those with sexual phobias or vaginal aversions, those who fear a loss of control over sexual urges and potential disastrous consequences, those with sexual deviations, and those who are concerned about aging.

LoPicollo's second category encompasses disturbances in the relationship between the man and his sexual partner: marital conflict, loss of attraction, poor sexual skills, fear of closeness, so-called mismatched couples, domineering partners with excessive demands, and an inability to fuse feelings of love and sexual desire. The effect of sexual dysfunction on a relationship is devastating and destructive in most cases and affects both partners (see chapter 6).

Predisposing, Precipitating, and Maintaining Factors

To better understand the various factors underlying psychogenic sexual dysfunction, we can apply, with some alterations, the model proposed by R. Basson et al. (2003), who divides predisposing, precipitating, and maintaining factors from contextual or immediate conditions that affect the outcome of a sexual encounter.

Predisposing factors involve sexual interest and desire, physical attraction, relationship dynamics, love and intimacy, and past life experiences. Constitutional factors, such as inborn anatomic, vascular, neurologic, and hormonal characteristics, as well as the individual's personality and temperament also play an important predisposing role in future patterns of sexual function and behavior.

Additional developmental factors, which include gender identity development; past painful, humiliating, or traumatic sexual experiences such as rape or abuse; and hormonal imbalance causing premature or delayed puberty, may contribute as well to the shaping of future sexual function or dysfunction.

Other important predisposing factors include religious, cultural, familial, social, and educational influences and personal views about sex.

Within that congenital and acquired physical and psychological framework, an individual may react negatively to certain precipitating factors, possibly impairing his or her sexual performance and desire. Among the most common psychogenic factors that may precipitate episodes of sexual dysfunction are performance stress, anxiety, depression, psychological disturbances, and relationship problems. These may all share a common pathophysiology such as a change in the inhibition of the parasympathetic nervous system, which normally stimulates the secretion of nitric oxide; alternatively, they may all lead to overactivity of the sympathetic nervous system, thereby constricting the penile arteries and precluding the development of normal erections.

Anxiety can produce cognitive distraction and reduce sexual arousal. Depression is generally linked with sexual dysfunction in a bidirectional way, which means that just as depression may be responsible for sexual impairment, the sexual dysfunction itself may also exacerbate the depression—especially with the use of certain antidepressive medications, which may worsen the sexual symptoms. Other precipitating factors include recent childbirth, infertility, divorce, financial problems, adultery, unemployment, a poor relationship, a traumatic sexual experience, loss of a beloved family member, issues related to homosexuality, poor personal hygiene, physical repulsion, or the partner's own sexual disturbances or ineptitude.

The most common factors in maintenance of sexual dysfunction beyond the original episodic disappointments are relationship disturbances, lack of intimacy, guilt feelings, performance anxiety, poor sexual education, and lack of communication. Other factors that play a pivotal role in the maintenance or persistence of sexual problems include lack of sexual experience, inadequate sexual stimulation, physical repulsion, fear of intimacy, psychiatric disorders, and loss of sexual chemistry.

I must emphasize the importance of a solid personal relationship and intimacy between partners for the success of their sexual relationship. The sexual disturbances of one partner may cause sexual problems for the other, compounded with loss of desire, feelings of guilt, anger, loss of self-confidence, and sometimes the urge to seek extramarital experiences or divorce. There may, of course, be some cultural and even gender discrepancies regarding the importance of love in sexual satisfaction and marital success, but in the Western world, the majority of men and women believe that deep affection, respect, emotional intimacy, and feelings of love are essential ingredients in optimal sexual pleasure and satisfaction.

Immediate contextual conditions that may affect the success of a sexual encounter include privacy, motivation and receptivity for sex, lack of sexual skills, environmental constraints, financial difficulties, physical or mental disease, emotional disturbance, anger, disrespect, ignorance or disregard of the partner's sexual preferences, premature ejaculation, and painful sexual intercourse.

PSYCHOLOGICAL THEORIES OF ETIOLOGY

Different schools of thought consider the psychological factors underlying male sexual dysfunction in a variety of ways (Hanash et al. 1994):

- Psychoanalytic theory proposes that during the period of psychosexual development (mental, emotional, and behavioral) between the third and fifth years of life, a boy wants to possess his mother, views his father as a rival, and fears that discovery of his feelings by his father would result in severe punishment. Therefore these sexual desires are repressed and kept subconscious as the child tries to identify with his father. This is called the Oedipus conflict. According to this theory, these early incestuous wishes and desires are carried into adulthood, along with fear and guilt, when the conflict is not successfully resolved in normal psychological development and maturation, and therefore a man's sexual disturbance or dysfunction is believed to be a defense against what he perceives as unacceptable childhood feelings. Psychoanalytic theory also contends that exposure to strict religious precepts condemning sexuality as sinful, shameful, and dirty eventually creates sexual difficulties. A psychiatrist of this school of thought would work with a patient to resolve these inner conflicts through interpretation and insight therapy.
- Learning theory contends that psychogenic sexual dysfunction is related to faulty learning and upbringing. For example, a boy who fears sexual expression because of the Oedipus conflict mentioned previously may later become impotent as a man; a boy who was punished for having sex may become impotent when he is exposed to a subsequent sexual experience; or a man who fears his sexual partner may learn to deal with that fear by avoiding sex. In other words, men who have negative experiences associated with sexual expression unconsciously try to avoid the anxiety engendered by such experiences, and ED or other sexual dysfunction can result.
- System theory, on the other hand, proposes that male sexual dysfunction is the result of a destructive relationship between the sexual partners. One of them may have a powerful urge to inflict pain, hurt, or humiliation on the other. Or, if a woman is feared to be "castrating" by her partner, or if her sexual needs are not met, her attitude and behavior can trigger insecurity, fear, and feelings of inadequacy in her partner, which can lead to anxiety and give rise to his ED.

PSYCHOLOGICAL DISTURBANCES AND ERECTILE DYSFUNCTION (ED)

Although there are legions of psychological causes for ED, four principal factors can be clearly identified: stress, anxiety, depression, and marital conflict.

Stress is how we react physically and emotionally to situations around us, how we respond to the changes, challenges, and unexpected events in our lives. Stress can be positive or negative. Positive stress helps us focus our energies, concentrate, and be productive—but it is positive only as long as we feel in control of the situation and as long as we can balance our stress with relaxation. Stress becomes negative when it is so constant, overwhelming, frustrating, or out of control that we cannot achieve the relaxation necessary for maintaining good mental and physical health. Uncontrolled stress can produce problems such as muscle tension, heart disease, stroke, high blood pressure, headache, backache, gastrointestinal problems, and sleep disorders; it can also cause either organic or psychogenic sexual dysfunction.

Anxiety's physiological manifestations, and the failure of the man's defenses to prevent or control it, may lead to sexual dysfunction that persists until the mental or intrapsychic conflicts producing the anxiety are resolved. Anxiety is a major cause of psychogenic ED. Although it is hard for women to understand it, many men are scared during the sexual act with fear of not being able to perform adequately and to match up with other men or to provide maximum pleasure to their partners, or to fail to develop or maintain an erection or to ejaculate quickly. This stress may preclude the expression of emotions and romantic feelings on his part, except maybe after the completion of a successful intercourse, when he feels relaxed. In contrast to women, who enjoy caressing and fondling all over their bodies for sexual excitation, a man needs reassurance about the quality of his erection, which is usually provided by direct caressing of the penis, which would also increase its firmness.

So-called performance anxiety, which differs from general anxiety, is also considered a major cause of psychogenic ED. In cases of performance anxiety and male sexual dysfunction, the man's concern about his sexual performance and fear of failure produces a state of anxiety, to which other intrapsychic conflicts are not significant contributors. (This distinction is important for the therapeutic approach.)

Depression is common to almost everyone. Most of us have sometimes felt down or blue, especially if we have had a particularly hard day or if we have been under pressure. It usually passes, though, and with a new day comes a brighter mood. Some people, however, cannot just snap out of it, and for them, depression can become a real and serious psychological disorder. It can also be a major cause of sexual disturbances, which in turn can worsen the depressive state.

Erectile failure produces psychological reactions in the male that cut across cultural, racial, and socioeconomic lines. A man's self-esteem, confidence, sense of manhood, and feelings of virility rely heavily on his erectile ability. A man who experiences the loss of an erection often feels that he is no longer a man. This can create frustration, loss of self-confidence, anger, humiliation, and shame—and any ensuing depression may well lead, unfortunately, to the development of ongoing ED.

Types of depression range from a mild passing condition to complete debilitation. Symptoms and signs can overlap, but some are unique to each type. Depressed people are usually blue, hopeless, irritable, and often tired. They tend to avoid social encounters, have trouble sleeping, and have little appetite. Generally, they have a decreased interest in sex. Sometimes they cry for no apparent reason and may even have thoughts of suicide. Just because a person has trouble sleeping, however, does not mean he or she is depressed. A psychologist looks for several symptoms that occur consistently over time before making a diagnosis of depression. Research also notes that men with ED and diabetes have a higher incidence of depressive symptoms and a negative health perception.

Depression affects all areas of an individual's life, including sexual interest and performance. Its treatment varies according to its nature and severity and may involve pharmacotherapy, psychotherapy, behavior modification, electroshock, or rational emotive therapy. Psychiatrists often prescribe antidepressant medications for patients with severe depression. Ironically, some of these medications may themselves cause sexual dysfunction.

Not surprisingly, research indicates that negative events, such as divorce, professional problems, financial difficulties, relationship difficulties, and marital conflicts, may contribute to psychogenic ED ("Proceedings of the First Latin American" 2003). Projections of self-doubt, inadequacy, and lack of trust carry over into a sexual relationship, and any negative perceptions that an individual carries about himself and/or his partner may contribute to poor sexual performance. A relationship charged with discord and deep conflict can be a major cause of male sexual dysfunction. Rejection of or by a partner is another common cause of ED. Conflicts occur in most close relationships, and marriage, as a long-term commitment, is not easy. Married couples often report reduced sexual desire, avoidance of sex, or erectile and ejaculatory problems.

Some reasons for conflicts in a marriage or relationship are unspoken expectations, inability to communicate effectively, jealousy, children and their demands, desire to change one's partner, self-image, appearance, obsession with performance, or simply the realities of life's day-to-day routine. Power struggle, sexual mismatch, dependency, distortions, financial problems, and lack of love, affection, and respect may all lead to sexual problems. Therapists and researchers often cite other causes for the development of sexual dysfunction within marriage, including alcoholism, infidelity, unfulfilled emotional needs, financial difficulties, and domineering or suspicious spouses. Any of these may lead to a marital breakdown, which in turn affects the couple's sexual attitudes and behaviors with each other.

Many therapists claim that the relationship disturbance is not so much because of the conflicts themselves, but rather because of the couple's lack of skills to handle them; that is, the real problem lies in the mode of interaction between the two people, rather than in either of them separately. An attempt by one partner, unskilled in effective communication, to bring about a behavior change in the other may severely strain the relationship. For example, a woman who wants to be flattered more by her husband may withhold sex until he complies. Her approach of punishing him to get her wish may be effective in the short term but ultimately harmful.

MISCELLANEOUS BEHAVIORAL AND PSYCHOLOGICAL CAUSES

Other psychosocial factors that may diminish sexual performance and desire include feelings such as fear, blame, shyness, and hostility; drug abuse or side effects of certain medications; and dissatisfaction with one's own body (as in cases of micropenis or marked obesity). A person's feelings about his or her body and physical appearance certainly influence the nature of his or her sexual activity. Embarrassment over the shape, size, or look of the genitalia or breasts, for example, interferes with successful fulfillment and enjoyment of the sexual act.

Some men are unable to abandon themselves to erotic pleasure and sexual feelings. A man's excessive self-observation and preoccupation with his sexual performance changes his role in sex to that of a spectator, rather than a full participant, which can impair his sexual functioning and may lead to erectile difficulties. Conflict about sexual identity, preference, and orientation may also impair sexual functioning.

A domineering or overly strict parent, a failure during early sexual encounters, and trying too hard to impress a partner are other contributors to psychogenic sexual dysfunction. In young men, homosexuality, religious orthodoxy, and sexual ignorance or misconceptions that may originate in a strict upbringing or misleading playground talk are among the most common psychogenic causes of ED.

Homosexuality

Homosexuality could actually be the subject of a whole series of books. Homosexuals often find heterosexual sex repulsive and totally unenjoyable. Granted, some bisexuals marry women and have a family. But it is not unusual that when a homosexual is married to a female, his heterosexual sexual aversion can become coupled with such profound guilt that a sexual dysfunction occurs in the marital relationship. That dysfunction may not exist during sexual encounters with men. Then again, guilt can induce such severe stress and anxiety that a homosexual man cannot achieve and/or maintain an erection with a male partner either.

Homosexuals are subject to all the physical and psychological causes of sexual dysfunction that heterosexuals are. Although no studies that I know of have been ever been conducted on the subject of male sexual dysfunction within the gay community, there is no reason to believe that homosexuality itself should significantly change the ratio of physical versus psychological causes of ED in homosexual males from that ratio in the heterosexual male population.

Religious Training and Family Background

Our future lives are shaped, to great extent, at an early age. We are the sum product of our environment and experiences. Some males raised under very strict religious rules tend to view sex as dirty, degrading, and morally wrong. In some cases, sex is tolerated only for procreation, and finding enjoyment and pleasure in sex is considered sinful. A large number of those men develop great anxiety and conflict between such deep-rooted moral beliefs and their normal, physiological, sexual urges. This condition often renders a man psychologically impotent and unable to engage in any sexual activity.

A young male who is raised by a single mother who is domineering and/or overly protective may lack an adult male figure with whom to identify. He may receive little or no motivation for sex or for gaining sexual experience. He may, based on his deep affection and attachment to his mother, project her image on all other females, hampering his ability to develop a normal sexual relationship. Without a strong male role model, a young male may lack self-confidence and could develop severe anxiety during any eventual sexual encounter, leading to erectile failure.

On the other hand, a young boy may feel incapable of ever living up to the expectations or image of a dominant, demanding, and strict father. In this situation, he can also lose self-confidence. As a man, he may develop deep anxiety when facing work, society, or sex. He may become an overachiever to prove himself. If he fails in any aspect, his anxiety deepens, stress develops, and his self-image suffers. It is not uncommon for chronic erectile failure to result.

Personality

Certain individuals are, by their personalities, more susceptible than others to psychogenic sexual dysfunction. These people often lack the proper psychological defenses that help in dealing with the stresses and strains of life in facing day-to-day problems. They may become depressed and withdrawn, feel helpless and anxious, and consider themselves to be inferior or failures. This sense of inadequacy, coupled with deep anxiety, can lead to sexual dysfunction.

The perfectionist, for example, sees performance as a yardstick by which to judge himself (and others). If he notices any change in his sexual ability, he becomes self-critical and loses his self-confidence and self-esteem; in trying to attack his problem aggressively and vigorously, he may develop more performance anxiety and fear of failure. The man who suffers from low self-confidence and constant self-doubts may interpret any problem in sexual performance as his fault. The compulsive worker or achiever, the overly independent, the placating individual, the intimidating or hostile individual, the obsessive, the suspicious, and the overly sensitive—all are among those whose personality traits make them susceptible to psychogenic ED.

Honeymoon ED

Some young men may experience total or partial ED on their wedding night or during their honeymoon. This may have a devastating effect on the man and his partner. In the past, the majority of these cases were attributed to psychological factors such as deep anxiety, excessive masturbation, ignorance, and fear of failure. Recent studies, however, have demonstrated the presence of vascular causes in about a third of these cases. Treatment with the phosphodiesterase type 5 inhibitor Tadalafil or the self-intracorporeal injection of Alprostadil or Trimix has been highly successful. (See chapters 11 and 12.)

Female Sexual Disturbances

A man's ED can sometimes be related to a lack of emotional or sexual intimacy with his partner, or perhaps to his partner's lack of sexual experience. Female sexual dysfunction, including poor libido, vaginismus, vaginal or intracoital disturbances or pain syndromes, urinary incontinence, comorbidities such as chronic systemic diseases, and overriding emotional or physical concerns, can contribute to her partner's ED, but these possible factors are often neglected during the evaluation of male patients (Singer AJ 2006).

Chapter Nine

DIAGNOSIS OF MALE SEXUAL DYSFUNCTION

Erectile dysfunction is a major healthcare issue and acts as a marker for other common major diseases. It therefore deserves attention, consideration, proper investigation, and appropriate treatment.

U.K. Management Guidelines for Erectile Dysfunction

In the past, most men suffering from sexual dysfunction were sent directly to psychiatrists. Some specialists still routinely refer all patients with apparent erectile dysfunction (ED) to a psychologist for diagnosis and treatment. However, general current opinion is that psychological consultation should be reserved for patients whose sexual troubles are suspected to be either purely psychogenic or a mixture of organic and psychogenic (see chapters 8 and 14). For instance, a happily married man who has no obvious emotional disturbances, a well-adjusted family situation, and an obvious physical cause for his ED need not see a psychologist for diagnosis.

Today's clinicians are gaining an ever better understanding of the physical and psychological causes of sexual dysfunction and have seen the advent of several new treatments. I now use a diagnostic algorithm relying on a comprehensive medical history, physical examination, and simple laboratory tests before initiating therapy. I reserve more elaborate (and invasive, and expensive) testing for exceptional cases. By first classifying my patient according to the etiology of his ED, I can then apply a goal-oriented therapy in what Dr. Adam Singer (2006) has termed a "shared informed decision" that is accepted and approved by the patient and his partner.

PREREQUISITES TO DIAGNOSIS AND TREATMENT

Before a man undergoes any medical tests and evaluations of the results, he must make a crucial decision based on his answers to the following questions:

What are his goals, anticipations, and expected outcome?
Is he seeking a doctor's opinion because he wishes to be treated?
Does he want to have tests run and find out their results?
Is he doing this for himself, or only to please his sexual partner?

If he decides he does indeed wish to pursue treatment, then he must understand that there is likely no single, simple solution to his ED. But although it may be complicated, a careful, thorough, accurate diagnosis of the ED's specific cause increases the chances of successful treatment. The process relies mainly on the man's understanding, cooperation, and sincere desire to be treated. Almost as important are his trust and confidence in his doctor and other team members, in full confidentiality at all times. His sexual partner, if any, must be considered a team member. It is ill advised for any man to undergo evaluation and treatment as a surprise for his sexual partner.

Before treating a man for a sexual dysfunction, we must also try to elucidate the causes of his problem and all the reversible risk factors such as smoking, low serum testosterone, alcoholism, drug addiction, obesity, lack of exercise, and certain medications. The elimination of these risk factors may lead to spontaneous recovery, without the need for any further treatment.

OVERVIEW OF THE DIAGNOSTIC PROCESS

For unknown millions of men, ED may be a temporary event in their lives. Other men, however, suffer more serious dysfunction from organic or combined psychological and physical factors that may be interrelated, and it can be difficult to tease these factors apart. Many men who were never able to develop or maintain a good erection, whose ED was thought to be psychogenic, have now been diagnosed with physical causes such as vascular or nervous system disorders. Perhaps as many as 80% or more of all cases of male sexual dysfunction have a physical basis. But men with ED, regardless of its cause, may develop emotional reactions to their problem that may contribute to its continuing or worsening.

As mentioned previously, all healthy men, regardless of age, develop spontaneous erections during sleep. Evaluating these erections helps differentiate, to a degree, psychological ED from physical ED. This assessment, however, cannot be the sole basis for diagnosis. Accurate diagnosis depends on review of the patient's medical, psychosocial, sexual, and familial histories; a proper physical examination; the results of some laboratory tests; and an open, frank discussion between the doctor and patient. The doctor needs to know when and how the sexual symptoms began as well as their character, nature, severity, and impact on the couple; document any previous illnesses or surgical procedures; and inquire about marital, familial, social, or professional factors that may contribute to the sexual dysfunction.

When a man with a sexual problem goes to see his doctor, his sexual partner should also be involved, if possible, in the process of diagnosis and treatment. The partner's attitude toward the problem should be carefully considered and discussed privately. The next step is to interview both parties together and separately. The doctor then compares the information received through questionnaires and separate interviews with both partners.

Following this interview process, the doctor conducts a complete physical exam, with special focus on the genitalia and the urinary, vascular, and neurologic systems. Normally, routine blood tests (fasting blood sugar level, lipid profile, serum testosterone, pituitary hormones, and thyroid function tests, for example) are then performed, depending on the patient's complaints, risk factors, and the results of the medical and sexual history and physical exam.

If the history, exam, and lab tests fail to reveal a definitive organic cause for the patient's ED, he may be treated with one of the phosphodiesterase type 5 (PDE-5) inhibitors or referred to a psychiatrist for psychological evaluation. But before going further, let me emphasize that it is extremely important to have the patient specify the exact nature of his sexual complaint to his doctor, whether it is truly ED, or premature or inadequate ejaculation, or lack of orgasm, because it is not uncommon for patients to get mixed up among them.

To ensure accurate evaluation of the sexual problem, especially in patients who do not respond to one of the PDE-5 inhibitors, such as Viagra, Cialis, or Levitra, or with whom there is a high suspicion of arteriogenic or veno-occlusive factors, intrapenile injection of a vasodilator may be attempted. This may rule out severe arterial occlusion or marked venous leakage, if the injection enables the patient to develop and maintain an erection for more than 10 minutes. If he fails to get an erection after the injection, a color penile Doppler ultrasound test may be performed, depending on the patient's age and history of trauma as well as on the possibility of performing surgery to correct a vascular lesion.

Doppler ultrasonography to assess blood flow velocity in the penile arteries before and after intrapenile injection of a vasodilator may suggest an arterial obstruction and/or an abnormal leakage through the penile veins (Brandstetter K et al. 1991). A peak velocity exceeding 35 centimeters (14 inches) per second excludes arterial obstruction. An end-diastolic velocity greater than 5 centimeters (2 inches) per second about 20 minutes after the injection may suggest a veno-occlusive defect. If a leak is indicated, injection of a contrast material into the corpora can confirm it radiographically (Bookstein JJ et al. 1988). In rare cases of suspected traumatic obstruction of a penile artery, pudendal arteriography (the injection of contrast material through the pudendal artery to visualize the penile vasculature) may be performed prior to attempting arterial bypass surgery.

Nowadays, various nonspecific treatments are often attempted on an empirical basis to help the ED patient achieve and maintain good erections for a sufficient time for sexual gratification, without addressing the major cause(s) of his dysfunction. For example, the majority of men with apparent ED are first prescribed a PDE-5 inhibitor (Viagra, Cialis, or Levitra) by their internists or family physicians without proper investigation. Only when they fail to respond to this form of therapy are they referred to urologists for further evaluation and treatment.

In certain complicated cases for which various types of therapy have been attempted and have failed, a team effort is often required to arrive at the correct diagnostic conclusion and effective treatment. The leader of the team is usually a urologist who specializes in treating male sexual dysfunction and is responsible for coordinating all the information gathering and medical testing. Other specialists may include marriage counselors, psychologists, psychiatrists, endocrinologists, neurologists, cardiologists, and social workers.

The urologist begins—and may complete—the diagnosis of ED by process of elimination. The best diagnostic tools are an open, frank, supportive, and complete interview (in most instances, of both the patient and his sexual partner) and a thorough physical exam. It is quite unfortunate that we physicians have become quite impatient in listening to the patient relate the history of his problems. Instead of using our ears and fingers to reach a diagnosis, we tend to rely on sophisticated equipment to make it on our behalf. It is often said that if we apply the art of careful listening, the patient himself may provide very important clues on which to make an informed, well-guessed diagnosis that may be confirmed later by laboratory tests.

It would be tragic to refer an ED patient with reversible vascular problems or low serum testosterone for psychiatric treatment, just as it would be highly undesirable to implant a penile prosthesis in a patient with purely psychogenic ED before attempting to solve the problem through psychotherapy. If, after the urologist's interview, exam, and necessary tests, purely psychogenic ED is strongly suspected, the patient and his partner are referred to a qualified psychiatrist or psychologist experienced in assessing and treating psychological sexual problems. If a combination of psychogenic and organic sexual dysfunction is suspected, the organic problems should be treated medically and the individual referred for concurrent psychological therapy. Consultation with a marriage counselor is important for all marital conflicts and discord.

For the correct diagnosis and proper treatment of ED, we should use the rifle and not the shotgun. We should not subject a man to a multitude of tests in the hope that one may yield a diagnostic clue. These tests can carry medical risks, may be quite annoying and stressful, and are sometimes very expensive. The interview and physical exam should help in selecting the most appropriate and cost-effective tests.

I should reemphasize that no further lab tests are warranted if a psychogenic or a particular organic cause is strongly suspected from the history and physical exam; if the patient is not a candidate for any particular treatment; or if he is unwilling to accept any form of invasive treatment (such as prostheses, vascular surgery, or intrapenile injections). In such cases, a hit-or-miss treatment approach involving oral medications or vacuum devices may be indicated— once the physician determines that sexual intercourse will not endanger the man's health. Other factors, such as the patient's age and comorbidities as well as the potential cost of treatment, are important considerations in determining the extent of the investigation.

CLINICAL INTERVIEW

The interview is the most important diagnostic tool for ED or other sexual dysfunction. It should be thorough and precise and should cover a sexual history, a medical history, and a psychosocial assessment. The involvement of the patient's sexual partner is important to corroborate and obtain more information about the dysfunction's history and course, any marital or familial problems, the priority of the sexual problem, the partner's attitude toward it, and the partner's own level of sexual interest and possible dysfunction. Interviewing the partner may change the patient's diagnosis and possible therapy in up to about 40% of ED cases.

Although it is time consuming, the physician or other health care professional needs to obtain answers to his or her diagnostic questions on a person-to-person basis. A good interviewer must be comfortable with face-to-face discussion of sexual matters. When it is necessary to put a patient or his partner at ease, or to get a point across, a good interviewer does not hesitate to use down-to-earth language. A good interviewer is not easily shocked and must assume that everyone does everything. It is not his or her place to apply values to the discussion, nor is it good practice, during the interview, to speak of normal or abnormal behavior.

At the very beginning, the patient must be questioned very precisely about the nature of his dysfunction to determine whether it is related to ED or another sexual problem. The patient's complaints, for example, may pertain to loss of sexual desire or to ejaculatory disturbances, which require different diagnostic testing and therapy. We need to know with some specificity about the problem's occurrence, duration, and effects on both the man and his partner, and any events that may have triggered it.

Examples of Interview Questions

The following can serve as examples of useful interview questions:

What is the nature of the problem?

Is an erection achieved and then lost?

Is the erection strong and rigid, or is it a soft and pliable erection?

Is the problem one of premature or retarded ejaculation?

Is there any erection at all?

When did the problem begin?

Under what circumstances did the problem begin?

Has the problem remained the same since it was first noticed, or have there been any changes? What are they?

What specific sexual activities did you engage in prior to the appearance of the problem?

What effect, if any, has the problem had on your sexual activities?

What is your frequency of masturbation, before and after the problem began? What is your level of satisfaction in terms of orgasm and ejaculation?

What is your frequency of intercourse, before and after the problem began? What is your level of satisfaction in terms of orgasm and ejaculation?

What is your frequency of oral sex, both as giver and receiver, before and after the problem began? What is your level of satisfaction in terms of orgasm and ejaculation?

What is your frequency of anal sex, both as giver and receiver, before and after the problem began? What is your level of satisfaction in terms of orgasm and ejaculation?

What is your frequency of the use of sexual aids or toys, before and after the problem began? What are they? What is your level of satisfaction in terms of orgasm and ejaculation?

What medications were you taking at the time the problem began? For what reason? What medications are you currently taking? For what reason?

Did you use illicit drugs before the problem began? What were they? What was the frequency of use? Were you using them at the time your problem began?

Do you smoke? How many cigarettes per day? How long have you smoked?

What was your alcohol consumption before the problem began? What is it now?

Do you currently experience morning erections? Are they rigid enough for intercourse? Do you use them for intercourse? For masturbation? How long do they last? Under what circumstances are they lost?

In your opinion, what is the major cause of your sexual problem?

When was the last time you had intercourse? Was your erection rigid? For how long could you maintain it?

Do you have strong sexual desire to engage in intercourse?

The interviewer will inquire specifically into past medical history as well as family, professional, economic, religious, and social background. The patient's relationship with his sexual partner will receive detailed attention, and the reactions of both people to the sexual dysfunction will be probed. Thinking on various social and sexual concerns will be explored, as the level and source of the patient's sexual knowledge will be important to the overall assessment.

QUESTIONNAIRES

As noted previously, it is best for clinicians to explore sexual questions directly with their patients, but a number of questionnaires specifically designed to assess sexual attitudes and functioning may be used in addition to the face-to-face interview.

In recent years, the Sexual Health Inventory for Men (SHIM) has been translated into more than 30 languages and used extensively worldwide. It has had great impact on the efficacy of ED management and has become a gold standard to measure treatment outcomes in clinical trials. It has also been adopted as a standard diagnostic aid to office screening for ED (Cappelleri JC, Rosen RC 2005). The SHIM consists of five items, with responses to each on a rating scale of 0 to 5. Scores higher than 21 indicate good sexual functioning, whereas 21 or less suggests possible ED, warranting further investigation. I want to emphasize, though, that this inventory should complement, not replace, clinical judgment and other standard measures for ED diagnosis. In a stable relationship, total scores classify ED as follows: 17–21 denotes mild ED, 12–16 denotes mild to moderate ED, 8–11 denotes moderate ED, and 1–7 denotes severe ED.

SEXUAL HEALTH INVENTORY FOR MEN

Each question has several possible responses. Circle the number of the response that best describes your own situation. Please be sure that you select one and only one response for each question.

Over the Past 6 Months

1. How do you rate your confidence that you could get and keep an erection?

   Very low = 1
   Low = 2
   Moderate = 3
   High = 4
   Very high = 5

2. When you had erections with sexual stimulation, how often were your erections hard enough for penetration (entering your partner)?

   No sexual activity = 0
   Almost never or never = 1
   A few times (much less than half the time) = 2
   Sometimes (about half the time) = 3

Most times (much more than half the time) = 4
Almost always or always = 5

3. During sexual intercourse, how often were you able to maintain your erection after you had penetrated (entered) your partner?

Did not attempt intercourse = 0
Almost never or never = 1
A few times (much less than half the time) = 2
Sometimes (about half the time) = 3
Most times (much more than half the time) = 4
Almost always or always = 5

4. During sexual intercourse, how difficult was it was to maintain your erection to completion of intercourse?

Did not attempt intercourse = 0
Extremely difficult = 1
Very difficult = 2
Difficult = 3
Slightly difficult = 4
Not difficult = 5

5. When you attempted sexual intercourse, how often was it satisfactory for you?

Did not attempt intercourse = 0
Almost never or never = 1
A few times (much less than half the time) = 2
Sometimes (about half the time) = 3
Most times (much more than half the time) = 4
Almost always or always = 5. (Cappelleri JC, Rosen RC 2005)

Another questionnaire, the Sexual Encounter Profile (SEP), is used extensively in clinical studies to assess ED treatment results. The most important items in the SEP (questions 2 and 3) pertain to the man's ability to achieve an erection firm enough for intercourse and to maintain it for a sufficient period until ejaculation and sexual satisfaction. An abbreviated tool called the Global Efficacy Questionnaire represents a description of whether a drug treatment has improved sexual function. Other questionnaires include the Psychological and Interpersonal Relationship Scales, the Drug Attribute Questionnaire, the Erectile Dysfunction Inventory of Treatment Satisfaction, the Treatment Preference Question, the Global Assessment Question, and others.

Although a patient's history and the absence of any noteworthy or known physical problem may suggest purely psychogenic ED, unfortunately, no single test can diagnose psychogenic, neurogenic, or myogenic (muscular) ED. These diagnoses are usually made by excluding organic causes through the use of several tests.

In, for instance, the case of a healthy man who abruptly develops ED unassociated with any medical or surgical condition, or other organic factors, and who reports significant psychosexual stress or marital conflicts preceding the onset of his sexual dysfunction, a psychogenic basis for his problem is highly suspected. This also applies to a man who can develop full erections during sleep, when waking in the morning, or during foreplay, masturbation, or sexual intercourse with a mistress, prostitutes, and/or others, but not with his wife or partner.

If a man, at least twice a week, has adequate erections on awakening, which last until he urinates, and has firm erections during foreplay and masturbation lasting for five minutes or more, his ED, in all likelihood, is psychogenic. On the other hand, a man who complains of poor or no erections during sleep and early morning or during masturbation and intercourse; who suffers from decreased penile sensations, which may make him lose his erection shortly after its development or before or during thrusting; or who exhibits a marked delay in achieving adequate erections is likely to have an organic cause for his erectile failure.

It is also important to question the patient regarding different risk factors such as past surgery and diseases including diabetes, hypertension, high cholesterol or serum lipids, vascular or cardiac conditions, and stroke; claudication in the lower limbs (pain on walking, with its disappearance at rest); trauma to the pelvis or to the perineal area (between the anus and the base of the scrotum); and smoking, drug abuse, and alcoholism, especially in young people.

If, from the history, a possible psychogenic or an organic cause is suspected, but the patient refuses any treatment or if medical or psychological considerations determine that there is nothing to offer him, no further tests are required. Only for patients who are willing to be treated, who are considered good candidates for various treatments, and who have a positive desire to resume a normal sex life is further testing warranted.

ROUTINE LABORATORY AND OFFICE TESTING

Although the lab tests selected may vary from one physician to another, the most common are blood tests, including a complete blood count, blood sugar, and hemoglobin A1C or a two-hour glucose tolerance test; serum testosterone (both total and free testosterone, especially in cases of decreased sexual desire; see chapter 16); and serum cholesterol, creatinine, urea, and triglycerides. If serum testosterone is low, serum prolactin is measured. Some specialists routinely order liver and thyroid function tests and other hormonal profiles. If pituitary disease is suspected, tests for serum follicular stimulating hormone and luteinizing hormone are ordered.

In young men, additional tests commonly employed in the initial screening for vascular problems include an assessment of penile blood flow with color duplex Doppler ultrasonography (Benson CB 1989). An electrocardiogram is usually ordered for all older men. A sickle cell profile and hemoglobin electrophoresis should be performed on all black men to rule out sickle cell disease or trait (sickle-shaped red blood cells but no other clinical manifestations of the disease), which may predispose them to priapism.

Some urologists may recommend testing for nocturnal penile tumescence (NPT; see the following discussion) to differentiate between psychogenic and organic ED, for medicolegal purposes, and for future documentation and follow-up of the patient. In some centers, a visual sexual stimulation test is performed, which consists of showing the patient a sexually stimulating movie of two consenting adults and measuring the occurrence and quality of his erections. I find this test especially helpful in cases of suspected psychogenic ED.

Nocturnal Penile Tumescence (NPT) Testing

The natural phenomenon of NPT is used to assess a patient's natural ability to develop erections during rapid eye movement (REM) sleep. As mentioned in chapter 4, healthy men develop one to five spontaneous erections per night, with an average of three (depending on age), which normally consume about 1.5 hours, or 20%, of the night's total sleep time. The average duration of each sleep erection is 27–38 minutes and decreases with age. It is assumed that if a patient's ED is purely psychogenic, his NPT test should reveal normal erections, with at least a 25-millimeter increase in circumference and with full rigidity for at least 10 minutes.

Conversely, it is assumed that the presence of any organic causes of ED may produce an abnormal NPT test result such as the absence of nighttime erections or a decrease in their intensity or frequency. However, NPT can also be abnormal in some cases of psychogenic impotence, in cases of neurologic disorder (such as spinal cord injury; see chapter 7), or in cases of so-called pelvic steal syndrome (when, during exercises involving the lower extremities, blood in the pelvis is shunted away from the penis toward the legs). Moreover, an NPT test may not always be a good indicator of a man's erectile potential in actual erotic circumstances.

Despite its limitations, NPT testing can demonstrate the partial or complete absence of erection in sleep or, alternatively, help a patient with psychogenic ED accept the etiology of his problem. Measurements of nocturnal tumescence and rigidity before and after therapy can also assist the physician in determining adequate titration (i.e., the smallest dose necessary) for intrapenile injections and provide objective documentation of the erectile failure's organic nature to insurance companies.

It is almost impossible for the patient to assess his own erections during sleep and quite difficult and impractical for his sexual partner to stay awake all night to measure the erections' number and quality, so several NPT tests have been devised.

Reliable tests of NPT are best conducted in the sleep laboratory of a hospital, clinic, or physician's office. These labs are equipped to perform electroencephalography, which records brain wave activity, and electro-oculography, which records eye movements and is used to correlate NPT with sleep quality and REM occurrence. Prior to testing, the patient must avoid anything that alters the sleep pattern (especially REM sleep) or causes insomnia, as it may affect the NPT test results. The most common test-contaminating factors are alcohol intake, heavy smoking, a large meal right before bedtime, exercise at night, and other stimulants such as coffee, tea, cola, chocolate (including cocoa), and sugar.

You may have heard that a patient's NPT can also be evaluated very simply—though not very precisely—at home, by using perforated stamps wrapped around the penis and sealed before the patient goes to sleep. If, in the morning, the perforations are broken, he may assume that a good erection occurred during sleep. Another method, called the snap gauge test, involves wrapping the penis in a Velcro fastener bearing three color-coded plastic bands designed to rupture at forces of 10, 15, and 20 ounces, which correspond to penile buckling and intracorporeal pressures. The degree of rigidity of the penis during erection correlates with the breakage of one, two, or three bands. Although these tests may sound like practical screening tools, they unfortunately do not provide sufficient information about the number, rigidity, and duration of nocturnal erections. They are not very accurate because of a high percentage of false-positive or false-negative results and are rarely used now.

A more sophisticated device, the Rigiscan (Dacomed), is composed of two components: a nocturnal penile rigidity and tumescence data-logging unit and a mini-computer that processes and prints the data. Two loops connected to the unit through a cable are placed at the base and tip of the penis before the patient goes to bed. During the night, the loops tighten every 15 seconds to measure penile circumference. The Rigiscan also measures the rigidity of any erection every 30 seconds. Recordings are made on three consecutive nights at home by the patient. He is instructed not to take naps, to avoid alcohol and drugs (except necessary prescription medications), and to refrain from sexual intercourse during the test period.

Following the test, the recording device is connected to a data processor, which downloads the information from the device's memory clip and prints the results of a 10-hour sleep period: number of erections per night, degree of rigidity of the penis during each erection, increase in the circumference of the penis, and duration of each erection. A good night's sleep without frequent awakenings, prolonged apnea (cessation of breathing), or excessive leg movement is necessary for accurate NPT results with sleep lab polysomnography or the Rigiscan.

Variations of the Rigiscan test include monitoring erections following intrapenile injections in a clinical setting, with the patient watching an erotic movie alone and without any disturbance that may lead to loss of the erection. A device similar to the Rigiscan, called the ART 1000, consists of two foam gauges, one to measure penile rigidity and the other to measure penile circumference, which are placed over the penis and connected to a computer that can store 27 hours of data collected over two consecutive nights.

Limitations of NPT Testing

Unfortunately, NPT tests are not very well standardized, foolproof, or always conclusive. It also should be stressed that sexually induced erections are different from spontaneous (reflexogenic) and sleep erections, so NPT testing may therefore be measuring different components of the erectile process. Although it can be very helpful, false-positive or false-negative results may occur in a substantial number of patients. For instance, a single, brief erection may give a false-positive result, suggesting psychogenic ED in a patient who actually suffers from organic ED. Furthermore, NPT may be absent or diminished because of the absence of REM sleep in spite of normal erectile physiology. Abnormality of the dorsal nerve of the penis, which carries sexual sensations, may cause sexual dysfunction despite normal NPT.

It has been reported that in 15% to 20% of patients with no organic causes for ED, no erections occur during REM (Lue TF 2000). This phenomenon can confuse the differentiation between psychogenic and organic ED. In addition, a few patients with psychogenic ED secondary to a condition such as severe depression may have an abnormal NPT result, whereas some with organic ED may have a normal NPT result.

Tests for NPT are generally reserved for specific cases and not used routinely. Most experts do not rely on NPT testing, except for medicolegal purposes or to convince a patient of the psychogenic nature of his impotence, because these doctors believe that the test does not represent the same type of sexual functioning experienced during intercourse. They believe that other tests, such as intrapenile injection of vasodilators, are more appropriate and accurate in reaching a correct diagnosis.

The greatest drawbacks in assessing NPT at home are lack of recorded information on the sleep pattern, lack of monitoring of the device's proper use, intentional falsification of the results by the patient, or even the device's effect on the patient's sleep pattern. Although the best way to test NPT is in a sleep lab, this poses several drawbacks as well. Spending two or three nights in a strange bedroom, with wires attached to your skull, eyes, and penis that in turn are connected to various monitors, and having an observer check your erections may not represent the ideal circumstances in which to enjoy a good night's sleep and perfect erections. In-lab NPT testing is also expensive and is not always readily available. It is, however, the best controlled and most accurate way to assess nocturnal erections.

A Crossroads: Treatment or Further Diagnostic Investigation

Depending on conclusions derived from the interview, histories, and physical exam, I may then begin the patient's treatment with the elimination of reversible factors such as smoking, obesity, low serum testosterone, certain medications, lack of exercise, or drug abuse, and if unsuccessful, proceed with one of the PDE-5 inhibitors (Viagra, Cialis, or Levitra). If that fails, I turn to the second line of treatment: intraurethral inserts of prostaglandin E1 (PGE1; alprostadil), a vacuum device, or intracorporeal injections of PGE1 or trimix.

If they all fail, and especially if the patient is young, I may check first regarding the proper use of these therapeutic methods, and then continue my search for a precise cause for his organic ED—provided, of course, that the patient is willing to undergo these tests and to accept further therapy if needed. I review all of the potential factors for his sexual dysfunction and then proceed with additional tests to reach a firm diagnosis, trying to rule out other possible organic and psychogenic causes for his ED and the reason for the failure of conservative therapies. Or I may propose the insertion of penile prostheses without further testing, especially if the patient is an older man and is willing to accept this aggressive treatment after a thorough discussion of its success rate, benefits, risks, possible complications, and cost.

VASCULAR TESTING

Several methods are used to check the integrity of the penile vascular system. These include the determination of penile blood pressure and blood flow using a Doppler ultrasound velocity detector or a pulse volume recorder. Ultrasonography is a simple, noninvasive test that may aid diagnosis, especially in young patients with a history of perineal trauma. A normal Doppler study in a young man usually suggests psychogenic ED. On the other hand, an abnormal Doppler study in an older man who has a history of vascular disease or takes various medications suggests a vascular or pharmacological cause for his ED. Other noninvasive adjunctive tests are also used.

Injections

Another method for differentiating between vascular and nonvascular ED involves direct intracorporeal injection of vasodilating chemicals such as PGE1 or papaverine, bimix (papaverine with phentolamine), or trimix (papaverine with phentolamine and PGE1). These substances directly dilate healthy penile arteries and sinuses, increasing blood flow to the corpora, resulting in engorgement, rigidity, and full erection. The Combined Intracavernous Injection and Stimulation (CISS) test may also be helpful in diagnosing vascular ED. The patient's self-stimulation in privacy after the injection (by watching an erotic movie with or without masturbation) may yield a better erectile response, especially if the injection elicits partial erection.

Following an intrapenile injection, the development of a rigid erection within 10–25 minutes and lasting more than 30 minutes may practically rule out any severe arterial or venous factors. Maintenance of a rigid erection for 30 minutes or more usually denotes the absence of venous leakage, an intact reflexogenic pathway for erections, and the lack of severe disease in the penile arterial system. However, a positive CISS test does not necessarily mean that penile arterial function is completely normal.

I should stress that any failure to develop an erection after the injection may be due to severe anxiety or absence of ongoing sexual stimulation. Also, when the injections are given in a clinical setting, the quality of the elicited erections is about 10% to 30% less than for the same injections used at home with better sexual stimulation, less distraction, and less embarrassment anxiety. Furthermore, these injection tests, which are still not standardized, may result in false-negative or false-positive results. Especially because they stimulate the cAMP and not the cGMP production in the corpora cavernosa.

In certain cases, when it is suspected that blood has been directed or shunted away from the penile arteries to the arteries of the lower extremities (steal syndrome), the patient is asked to perform knee-bending exercises during erection, without any injections. If a steal or shunt of blood is present, he will lose his erection during these exercises. If the penile arteries are clogged or severely diseased, or if there is abnormal venous leakage, there will not be enough arterial or sinusoidal dilation for an erection to occur, or if an erection does occur in such a case, it will be lost quickly following an intrapenile injection.

In almost all other organic or psychogenic conditions, intracorporeal injections result in normal erections. The idea behind penile injection testing is that the adequacy or inadequacy of arteries and sinuses can be checked while bypassing all the other factors that may affect them. It assesses the integrity of the intrapenile arteries and sinuses and their ability to dilate under the influence of the vasodilating substances injected directly into the corpora. These chemicals are also used to treat patients with ED for whom oral pharmacological therapy is ineffective (see chapter 12).

If I strongly suspect significant vascular disease from a young patient's history, physical exam, and the previously mentioned noninvasive tests, I proceed with additional tests to confirm the diagnosis and give a clearer picture of the penile arteries' anatomy and possible problems.

Imaging

Some physicians routinely check the blood flow and blood pressure of the penile arteries with a Doppler ultrasound during the initial physical exam of any patient presenting with possible ED. The penile blood pressure value is divided by the systemic blood pressure value to obtain the penile blood pressure index (PBI). If the PBI is lower than 0.6, penile vascular disease is highly suspected; when the index is 0.6–0.75, it is suggestive, but not diagnostic, of diseased penile arteries; and a PBI over 0.75 usually denotes a healthy penile vascular system.

Another noninvasive method called plethysmography, which provides a paper record of the pulse volume in the penile arteries, has been largely replaced by the more accurate duplex ultrasonography and pulsed Doppler analysis. This test is performed before and after the intracorporeal injection of a vasodilator such as papaverine or PGE1. It demonstrates the diameter of the arteries passing through the corpora cavernosa, which should increase following the injection, if the arteries are intact. Simultaneously, the Doppler sonogram measures blood flow through these arteries. Blood pressure within the cavernous arteries may also be checked and recorded before and after the injection. If blood flow in the central cavernosal arteries is less than 25–30 milliliters per second after the injection, arteriogenic ED is strongly suspected. Furthermore, if end diastolic pressure is over 7 millimeters of mercury, veno-occlusive disorder is strongly suspected. Unfortunately, this is a costly and operator-dependent test. Results can also be abnormal in some patients with psychogenic ED, due to severe anxiety during the test.

Radioisotope imaging with a technethium scan or MRI to check the integrity of the penile vascular system can be used as well. If this imaging result is abnormal, a venous leak or a combination of arterial and venous disease may be suspected and further tests performed. The Free University of Berlin in Germany has also added determination of the oxygen content of the corpora to the diagnostic armamentorium for ED.

Arteriography and Microsurgery

If the penile vascular system is found to be abnormal, the patient is younger than 50, with no history of generalized vascular disease, heavy smoking, or diabetes, and he has a history of trauma to the perineal area or genitalia, I may conduct further testing for an obstruction of the pudendal or penile arteries— provided that he is willing to undergo an arterial treatment technique (such as balloon dilation or microsurgical reconstruction) if an obstruction is found.

The most accurate test for this purpose is selective pudendal arteriography. In this procedure, a contrast dye is injected into the pudendal artery, coloring it and the off-branching penile arteries so the radiologist can visualize them. Sometimes visualization is further enhanced by intra-arterial injection of a vasodilator. This rather invasive test reveals the anatomy of the pudendal and penile arteries and the nature of their disease, helping the surgeon select the best surgical approach. Unfortunately, in some cases, it is difficult to correlate the defect seen in this arteriograph with the patient's specific functional problem.

If a unilateral or bilateral obstruction or narrowing of the pudendal or penile artery is discovered, the radiologist may perform balloon dilation of the less-affected side, or the surgeon may bypass the obstruction by joining (anastomosing) an epigastric artery from under the abdominal rectus muscle to either the dorsal penile artery or vein to ensure good blood flow to the penis. Before this procedure is performed, the patient is informed about all aspects of the surgery and the chances (about 20% to 60%) of long-term success. The ideal candidate for such a revascularization procedure is a healthy, nonsmoking young man who has no diabetes or arteriosclerosis, with a traumatic occlusion of a pudendal or penile artery. The surgeon's expertise in this procedure is of great importance for a successful result. The operation, if successful, helps the patient recover natural erections.

Some men with ED but normal cavernosal arterial function are more likely to be suffering from other problems such as fibrosis and destruction of the lining of the cavernosal sinuses or the smooth muscle, thinning of the tunica albuginea, dysfunction of the ischiocavernous muscles surrounding the corpora, or endocrinological conditions such as diabetes. For certain patients with severe diabetes and atherosclerosis, a biopsy of the cavernous tissue for further examination may be indicated, but this is rare.

Tests for Venous Leakage

There are a substantial number of men with organic ED, especially in the over-50 group, whose primary problem is a leak from the penile venous system during erections. For these men, blood flows through the penile veins at such a rate that not enough blood is trapped within the penis to cause engorgement and erection. It is now believed that the majority of venous leakage cases are associated with incomplete relaxation of the cavernous smooth muscle due to smooth muscle disease (diabetes, hypertension, high cholesterol, etc.), psychogenic sexual dysfunction, or weakening of the tunica; more rarely, a leak may be congenital or acquired. Increased inflow through the arteries and decreased outflow through the veins are necessary to develop and sustain a rigid erection.

A venous leak can be demonstrated, or even strongly suspected, if, during a natural erection or following an intracorporeal vasodilator injection, it becomes difficult to maintain the erection by continuous infusion of saline solution into the corpora. If the erection cannot be maintained with a small volume of infusion, or if the intracorporeal pressure drops rapidly and the erection is lost when the infusion is stopped, a venous leak is likely. A cavernosography, in which dye is injected into the corpora cavernosa to visualize the vasculature, may show the leaking vessels.

During testing for venous leakage, it is important to ensure that the smooth muscles of the corpora are completely relaxed, with a full erection, to avoid a false-positive result. There is still no consensus on established techniques, standards, and data norms for these tests, so their results should be cautiously interpreted. Furthermore, injection of hyperosmolar (highly concentrated) contrast material may cause severe corporal inflammation and scarring, possibly even leading to ED.

The identification of such a leak and its subsequent surgical repair could yield minimal success in a few selected cases, although results have been disappointing in the majority of cases on long-term follow-up. If the site and extent of a venous leak can be found, it can be treated by perineal exercises, intrapenile injections, constrictive rings, or vacuum devices. It can also be treated surgically by ligating the abnormal vessels, or by sclerotherapy, which consists of injecting sclerosing solutions into the abnormal veins to scar and obstruct them.

The success rate is, however, very low for most of these methods: in the vicinity of about 20% to 30%, which may, in selected rare cases, reach about 50% to 60%, depending on the veins and procedures involved. Surgery for venous leakage has been largely abandoned and is very seldom performed, especially because such leaks are generally attributed nowadays to diseased corporeal tissue and an inability of the vascular sinuses to dilate properly for normal obstruction of the leaking veins.

NERVOUS SYSTEM TESTING

Before reaching a conclusive diagnosis, I check the integrity of all systems involved in the erectile process. I have so far discussed the various tests used for the vascular, endocrine, and genital systems. That leaves the nervous system, which comprises the brain, spinal cord, and penile peripheral nerves, and for our purposes may also include the hypothalamus and pituitary gland.

If I suspect a neurologic disease from the patient's medical history, and if a careful physical exam reveals sensory or motor changes affecting the cranial nerves, sensory changes, reflex changes, or other neurologic signs, I may conduct additional neurologic examination to confirm the diagnosis and localize the site and extent of the lesion. I start with simple, readily available tests and then proceed with more complex testing under the supervision of a neurologist.

Penile biothesiometry, a simple and commonly used sensory test, assesses the perception threshold of the penile skin. The examiner places an electromagnetic vibrator on the shaft of the patient's penis and controls the amplitude of the vibrations. The patient informs the examiner of the first sensation he notices, as vibration amplitude is slowly increased or decreased.

Biothesiometry provides information regarding the integrity of the penile dorsal nerve and normal afferent penile sensation (i.e., signals traveling from the nervous system to the penile nerves). It may be used as a screening test in all potential ED patients. If there is no history of neurologic disease and the biothesiometry result is normal, neurogenic ED may generally be ruled out.

More advanced tests performed by a neurologist or neurophysiologist check the conduction time of neural impulses traveling along the nervous system. Electromyography (measuring electrical activity) of the cavernous muscles before and during erection, for example, provides information regarding the integrity of the efferent penile neurologic process (i.e., sensory signals traveling from the penile nerves to the nervous system). But if biothesiometry is abnormal and a neurologic disease is suspected from clinical findings, additional neurologic tests are rarely used to diagnose more specific neurogenic factors in ED.

Unfortunately, there is still no accurate test for the integrity of the autonomic nervous system or the sympathetic and parasympathetic nerves that are directly involved in erection and ejaculation. Cavernosal electromyography has been reported to be helpful for this purpose, but studies are needed to confirm its usefulness. Cavernosometry is contraindicated, however, for patients treated with monoamine oxidase inhibitor antidepressants because the combination could precipitate a severe hypertensive crisis (i.e., an extreme increase in blood pressure). Furthermore, this test, like pudendal arteriography, is not well standardized, as data norms are lacking, and its interpretation is not very accurate.

If a spinal cord problem, such as a herniated lumbar disk or tumor, is suspected, a spinal MRI or a myelogram (radiology of the spine following injection of contrast medium into the cord's subdural space) is performed to confirm the diagnosis and delineate the site of the disorder.

Other neurologic tests exist but are seldom used outside of research purposes. Single potential analysis of cavernous electric activity, pioneered in

Germany, also records the electrical activity of the cavernous tissue. Its preliminary results in differentiating between organic and psychogenic ED are encouraging. It may be particularly helpful for diagnosing neurogenic ED.

LIMITATIONS OF DIAGNOSIS

In principle, a treating physician can expect good results if he or she is able to make an accurate diagnosis and apply a specific treatment to the identified cause of the ED. In some cases, doctors still cannot pinpoint the causes of a sexual dysfunction, even after performing some or all of the tests described herein. Unfortunately, normal values for most of these tests are not yet precisely known, nor is their exact accuracy in reaching a precise diagnosis. But at least these tests may provide some objective means to differentiate between various etiologic factors in selected cases, especially in young patients. They may also help in selecting the most appropriate mode of treatment to obtain the best results and avoid unnecessary and sometimes dangerous procedures.

I should, however, emphasize again that most of these tests are rarely employed nowadays, and that the majority of experts rely on medical and sexual histories, physical examination, and routine laboratory testing to reach an ED diagnosis and start treatment with one of the PDE-5 inhibitors. Furthermore, some physicians—especially internists, general practitioners, and even some urologists—start treatment without any testing, arguing the non-cost-effectiveness of testing and its noncontribution to initial management of ED. This attitude, however, may lead to missing some important diseases that underlie the ED and may produce other major complications if left undiagnosed and untreated.

A new noninvasive test using a tissue oximeter has been used to check the degree of oxygenation of the penile tissue in the flaccid and erect state before and after the intrapenile injection of vasodilators in men with or without ED. This technique may prove important to checking the degree of hypoxia in the cavernous tissue in men with ED (Padmanabhan P, McCullough AR 2006). In certain cases of poor penile oxygenation, oximetry may be valuable for proper diagnosis and management.

In the future, more precise and standardized tests of the integrity of the penile smooth muscle and the tunica, the level of the neurotransmitters in the corpora, and any pathology affecting the lining of the vessels and sinuses will yield more accurate diagnosis and better choice and application of therapy.

Chapter Ten

CONSERVATIVE TREATMENT OF ERECTILE DYSFUNCTION: CRITICAL CONSIDERATIONS

Love is the answer, but while you are waiting for the answer, sex raises some pretty good questions.

Woody Allen

To obtain the best results from treatment of erectile dysfunction (ED), its early identification, diagnosis, and management are of utmost importance. This chapter outlines some critical points in dealing with this process. Chapters 11–14 then provide a comprehensive review of all the therapeutic modalities used for ED.

The treatment recommended for, and chosen by, a man with ED should be as conservative and simple as possible and individualized on the basis of his diagnosis and specific needs. After a thorough discussion of all options, the selection of an ED treatment is best accomplished as a shared decision between the patient and his partner, according to their expectations and preferences, and the treating physician or therapist, based on the clinician's experience and judgment and on evidence-based, clinical results of the various modes of therapy available.

The treatment of ED was revolutionized by the introduction of the phosphodiesterase type 5 (PDE-5) inhibitors: Viagra in 1998, and Levitra and Cialis in 2003. These oral medications come close to fitting the definition of the ideal treatment for ED that I proposed in the *Journal of Urology* (Hanash KA 1997). They are easy to use, efficacious, safe, dependable, and acceptable to many patients and their sexual partners and have only a low incidence of minor side effects. On the other side of the coin, however, they are expensive, averaging about \$8–\$10 per tablet. Also, to a large number of men and/or their partners, these drugs represent an artificial means of producing erections, which may not be acceptable to them.

Instead of, or in addition to, taking a PDE-5 inhibitor, ED treatment may consist of one or more of the following:

Changing or discontinuing certain medications
Discontinuing use of drugs, alcohol, and/or anabolic steroids
Cessation of smoking and any other tobacco use
Weight loss and exercise
Testosterone supplementation
Sex therapy
Behavioral therapy
Psychotherapy
Education and counseling, including marital counseling
Specific instructions for more effective sexual stimulation
Elimination of sexual inhibitions
Elimination of sexual misconceptions, taboos, and myths
Creams or ointments
Vacuum devices and/or constriction rings
Penile injections
Urethral inserts of prostaglandin E1 (PGE1; alprostadil)
Surgical improvement of the blood supply to the penis
Correction of penile venous leakage
Prosthetic penile implants
Herbs and other natural products

Several experimental substances and techniques are also of more than passing interest.

Treatment for ED generally starts with the simplest methods. The primary line of conservative treatment is an orally administered PDE-5 inhibitor. If the medication fails (which occurs in about 30% to 50% of cases), reinstruction as to its proper administration or switching to another PDE-5 inhibitor may be attempted. If the patient again experiences treatment failure with these drugs, or refuses them, the second line of conservative treatment is attempted. This includes a vacuum device, intraurethral inserts, intracorporeal injections, and some natural products and herbs. These treatments may be tried in combination with each other or with a PDE-5 inhibitor. If the patient continues to experience treatment failure, a penile prosthesis could then be inserted, or, in selected cases, investigation of the penile vasculature may be warranted for the consideration of other surgical corrective techniques.

Keep in mind that PDE-5 inhibitors, vacuum devices, intraurethral inserts, intracorporeal injections, and penile prostheses do not cure the original disease or disorder causing the ED. They merely help the man achieve an erectionlike state rigid enough for successful penetration, intercourse, and sexual satisfaction.

An analogy: it is like using a hearing aid for a severely hearing-impaired patient whose diseased or damaged auditory nerve is incurable; the device simply allows the individual to override the basic problem that still exists.

DIAGNOSIS AND TREATMENT OBJECTIVES

Again, the best treatment for any case of ED should be as simple and noninvasive as possible, effective, well accepted, and planned by the patient and his partner, according to their particular emotional and physical circumstances. Ideally, it should aim at the cause of the ED—and, if possible, cure it—with a high rate of success and a low rate of complications. At the very least, it should restore the man's sexual capability, have few or no side effects, and be affordable.

Choosing a Doctor

The man seeking diagnosis and treatment must choose the clinician(s) in whom he has the most confidence to give him the best results. No man who suspects he has ED, or has been previously diagnosed with ED, should proceed with any form of ED treatment before consulting a physician with expertise in this area—preferably a urologist—for a complete medical evaluation to detect any medical conditions causing or contributing to his sexual dysfunction.

In choosing a physician and/or therapist, a patient must focus on the clinician's experience, knowledge, skills, character, qualifications, objectivity, past results, and bedside manner as well as the scientific methods he or she applies to the problem and the confidence he or she instills. It is always advisable, if possible, to check with other patients who have been treated by the various physicians or therapists being considered. Such patients can offer valuable insight into the clinicians' skills and the results and satisfaction that can be expected.

The patient must be alert to the so-called specialist who wants to impose opinions on him and be wary of anyone who wants to try nonapproved herbs, potions, lotions, or devices, or who claims expertise in some obscure and unconventional procedure. He must keep away from any physician who refuses to discuss the problem, answer all his questions, or provide all the information he needs on the full range of available treatment options. And of course, he must ensure that he does not fall into the hands of a quack promising a magic pill or potion as a sure and fast cure for his sexual dysfunction.

These remarks carry a connotation of "buyer beware"—and indeed, there is a perception on the part of many people, both inside and outside the medical community, of an ethics problem in the so-called ED trade. Some scientists and clinicians may be too eager for personal recognition and/or financial reward. A researcher, for example, can shade the results of a study into a conclusion that has no basis in factual evidence, or a doctor can apply undue pressure on a patient to undergo an expensive surgical procedure, when a less expensive therapy could yield results as good or better and without the long-term risks and complications.

A man seeking help for a sexual problem must insist on being fully educated about the anatomy and physiology of the sexual organs, the details of normal sexual mechanisms, and the causes of his dysfunction. He must also satisfy himself as to the expertise and general motivation of his doctor or therapist before agreeing to any diagnostic testing and/or treatment. If a patient is not fully confident in the treating clinician, or if he has any lingering doubts about the proposed treatment, he would be wise to seek other medical opinions.

Obtaining a Diagnosis

For the greatest likelihood of success, ED's treatment should be tailored as much as possible to its medically evaluated etiology. Diagnostic examination may also reveal other diseases such as severe cardiovascular conditions, which—in addition to being life threatening—may necessarily prevent or delay the use of certain ED treatments.

A substantial number of men, however, are subjected to a shower of tests and aggressive therapy for presumed ED when their problem, misdiagnosed during their interview, may actually be lack of sexual desire or premature ejaculation. As detailed in chapter 7, the proper diagnosis can be made by a thorough, careful history backed up by a physical exam and confirmed by simple tests. Sometimes, all that a man with ED really needs is reassurance, some simple therapeutic methods to improve his overall health and well-being, and good sex education to eliminate myths, misconceptions, and sexual inhibitions. For men who only require these modes of treatment, a battery of sophisticated, expensive tests is unwarranted, and may even be counterproductive.

Many physicians believe that in cases of suspected ED, extensive testing is neither medically rewarding nor cost-effective, and they prefer to skip it. Often, after diagnosing a patient's ED with a thorough history, physical examination, and a few basic blood tests, finding no medical contraindications, and obtaining the patient's consent, the physician initiates pharmacotherapy with one of the PDE-5 inhibitors.

A word of caution is appropriate here: ordering PDE-5 inhibitors on the Internet, soliciting them from friends or pharmacies without prescriptions, or using a nonapproved knockoff without prior medical consultation is foolish and ill-advised. These widespread practices may lead to dangerous and sometimes fatal complications and should be totally prohibited.

Importance of Accurate Diagnosis for Proper Treatment Choice

Sam is a 45-year-old man who sought medical help for ED of some 12 months' duration. The urologist, after interviewing Sam and performing a physical exam (mainly on the genitalia), ordered blood tests for sugar, testosterone, and prolactin levels. When the test results showed no abnormalities, the urologist prescribed Viagra, but Sam had no positive response to the drug. On a follow-up visit, because Sam's condition had not improved, he was advised to undergo surgery for the insertion of a penile prosthesis.

Sam rightly decided to seek a second opinion, so he consulted a second urologist, one with extensive experience in sexology. On interviewing him, this physician discovered a significant history of professional and marital problems that corresponded to the time Sam's sexual difficulties began. The physical exam and routine blood tests were normal, and intracorporeal injection of PGE1 in the office elicited good erections. He referred Sam to a psychiatrist and a marriage counselor, who confirmed the diagnosis of psychogenic ED, and Sam was successfully treated with sex therapy.

Perhaps no harm would have been done if Sam had initially agreed to a penile prosthesis, and at any rate, he would have had the capability of erection on demand; penile prostheses have high success rates. Nevertheless, there are specific indications and contraindications for their use, and they should be reserved as the last treatment option when all other therapeutic modalities have failed. The surgical insertion of prostheses carries inherent risks, possible medical and mechanical complications, physical and psychological stress, and high cost.

Choosing a Treatment

It is important to realize that only a few of the available treatment options can fully restore natural erections. Often, a therapeutic modality will help a man with ED achieve firm erections for successful intercourse, but without addressing the root cause(s) of his sexual dysfunction or providing a permanent solution. Moreover, those erections may not totally resemble his normal erections in their quality, spontaneity, degree of rigidity, and duration. The PDE-5 inhibitors, for example, are sexual enhancers, not promoters; as such, they have no effect at all in producing an erection without sexual stimulation, and they do not increase sexual desire.

But this does not imply that ED is incurable or that "once impotent, always impotent," as some therapists erroneously suggest. In fact, for about 30% of carefully selected patients, simple behavioral measures such as smoking cessation, daily exercise, a balanced diet, reduced obesity and serum cholesterol, moderated alcohol intake, avoidance of illicit drugs and steroids, discontinuation of some medications, relief of anxiety and stress, or even knowledge of proper sex techniques may be sufficient to recover normal sexual functioning, without the need for further treatment. A recent study covering 401 men with ED followed for a period of nine years from 1987–1989 to 1995–1998, and up to 15 years (2002–2004), with no treatment in the Massachusetts Longitudinal Aging Study revealed some interesting and unexpected findings. While about 33% of men with minimal or moderate ED exhibited ED progression, about 32%, 14%, and 31% of men with minimal, moderate, and complete ED, respectively, recovered full sexual potency. Weight loss, cessation of smoking, and improvement of overall health were the most important factors involved in the remission of ED and/or delaying its progression (Travison TG et al. 2007). In certain other cases, specific medical measures, such as supplementing low hormone levels, repairing a herniated disk, or bypassing an arterial occlusion, may restore normal erections.

As you can see, it is extremely important for the patient to look at his own case for reversible factors, which, if corrected with professional help and personal willpower, may help him regain full sexual ability without the need for artificial and expensive therapeutic interventions. All treatment options and their success rates, risks, benefits, possible complications, and cost should be explained to him (and his partner) by the treating physician.

Treatment with PDE-5 inhibitors is generally effective in about 70% of patients with ED. If it is not, the patient is usually referred to a urologist, who will assess the cause of the failure and likely prescribe other nonaggressive options such as a vacuum device, intraurethral inserts, or intracorporeal injections. If all of these options are unsuccessful, and after obtaining the patient's approval, the urologist proceeds with surgical insertion of a penile prosthesis, unless the patient's choice and/or other medical considerations indicate a different course of treatment. It is important to understand that surgery solely for restoring sexual function is elective and not a matter of life or death.

No treatment for ED, conservative or aggressive, should be undertaken if the patient is not fully convinced of its necessity and efficacy. If he is not ready to accept all the potential side effects or complications of any recommended form of treatment, or if the treating physician or therapist cannot reasonably assure his expectations of the anticipated results, he should not proceed with it.

It is also highly desirable that the selected treatment be fully acceptable to the patient's partner, with whom he should candidly and objectively discuss any proposed treatment beforehand. A man should never, under any circumstance, hide his treatment from his partner, especially if he has chosen injections, a vacuum device, or a penile prosthesis. The later surprise may only aggravate any existing sexual and relationship problems and compound the man's (or couple's) dysfunction.

Cautionary Tales

Some treatment methods are dangerous and may be unnecessary when other options exist. As I have stressed, it is always better and safer to treat the patient with the simplest methods first and, if they are unsuccessful, to proceed gradually with the more invasive ones.

For example, the insertion of a penile prosthesis in a young man with psychogenic ED is generally inadvisable, as it is likely to result in postoperative emotional problems, poor satisfaction, worsening of the psychological disorder, and litigation. In rare cases, a prosthesis can be implanted if all other therapeutic options have failed, and following counseling and a thorough psychiatric assessment and psychotherapy by an expert psychiatrist, who should advise and approve the surgery.

It is critical for any penile prosthesis candidate to understand that its insertion permanently destroys much of the cavernous tissue inside the penis, making other modes of treatment inapplicable in the future, and that it may also shorten the penis. For illustration, consider a patient with purely psychogenic ED who is treated initially with a penile prosthesis. If his psychological problems are later successfully managed and he wants the prosthesis removed, he will, in all likelihood, be left with partial or complete organic ED because of the tissue destruction that occurred with the device's insertion—and any further treatment will generally be unsuccessful.

Now, consider a man who has a severe generalized vascular disease affecting his penile arteries and who has a negative response to intracorporeal injections of vasodilators. He may need a more thorough evaluation of his penile vascular system, especially if he did not respond to treatment with PDE-5 inhibitors and other noninvasive therapies. Depending on his age and underlying vascular status, this patient might ultimately require a penile prosthesis or vascular surgery.

Treatment for the diabetic man with ED who does not have severe vascular, neurologic, hormonal, genitourinary, or psychological disease begins with simple, safe pharmacotherapy. However, the patient's diabetes may not necessarily be the root of his sexual problem; other organic or psychogenic factors may actually be the primary causes. If he is taking antihypertensive drugs such as diuretics, or beta-blockers such as propanolol, both of which are known to cause ED, other antihypertensives can be substituted, and his nephrologist may switch him to calcium channel blockers, alpha-blockers, or vasodilators. On the other hand, if no definitive organic or psychogenic causes are elicited by a thorough evaluation, the patient could be prescribed one of the PDE-5 inhibitors and instructed to stop smoking (if he is a smoker), lose weight, and exercise.

In all older men, treatment with testosterone is not recommended and is rarely helpful, except for certain men with significantly low levels of testosterone (especially free serum testosterone; see chapter 16); even for some of these patients, hormone replacement may not yield good results, and other therapeutic options, such as the addition of a PDE-5 inhibitor, should be tried. Furthermore, testosterone treatment may carry side effects such as a possible flare-up of an occult prostate cancer, water and sodium retention, abnormal lipid metabolism with elevated serum cholesterol, liver dysfunction, and increased red blood cells, which may lead to vascular occlusion.

MANAGING ERECTILE DYSFUNCTION SUBSEQUENT TO PROSTATE CANCER TREATMENT

Prostate cancer is the most common malignant tumor in men older than 50 and the second most common cause of mortality, after lung cancer, in this age group in the United States and most of Western Europe. Its management depends on the tumor's grade and stage; the patient's age, existing comorbidities, and initial level of serum prostate-specific antigen (PSA); and whether the cancer has spread beyond the prostate. As with all ED patients, treatment selection is a decision shared by the urologist and the patient who has been fully educated about all the therapeutic options, success rates, benefits, hazards, adverse reactions, and complications.

For nonadvanced cancer confined strictly to the prostate, the treatments most commonly employed are watchful waiting, radical prostatectomy, external radiation therapy, or brachytherapy (insertion of radioactive seeds in the prostate). For advanced localized cancer, radical prostatectomy, possibly with hormonal therapy or with combined radiation and hormonal therapy, is the standard of management. In a case of diffuse (widespread) metastases, hormonal therapy using GnRH agonists or antagonists, antiandrogens, female hormones, or castration is considered the treatment of choice (without prostatectomy).

The incidence of ED after radical prostatectomy varies from 20% to 100%, depending on the patient's age, erectile function prior to surgery, surgical preservation of the neurovascular bundles (the nerves and vessels that supply the corpora cavernosa), comorbidities (such as diabetes, hypertension, or atherosclerosis), the stage of the tumor, and the surgeon's experience. For patients whose prostate cancer was treated with external radiation therapy, which causes the penile vasculature's lining to thicken, the incidence of posttreatment ED gradually increases with time, reaching 50% to 80% after three to five years. Brachytherapy is associated with the lowest rate of posttreatment ED at 10% to 30%.

After prostatectomy, a patient may take up to two years to recover his erectile ability, with or without PDE-5 inhibitors or other nonaggressive therapy for his ED. Several clinical studies, however, have demonstrated that sexual rehabilitation with nonaggressive treatments beginning a few weeks after surgery may help many of these patients regain their potency much sooner and with a higher rate of success.

In one study of patients with one or both neurovascular bundles preserved but with persistent ED two years postoperatively, each of the PDE-5 inhibitors (Viagra, Cialis, and Levitra) yielded encouraging results when used daily or on demand prior to sexual intercourse. About 60% to 70% of the men taking the medication reported improved erections, compared to about 24% for placebo. Furthermore, about 60% to 70% of the men who had erectile improvement regained the ability to develop an erection firm enough for penetration and maintained long enough for successful intercourse—particularly when low-dose (25 mg) Viagra was administered nightly for up to 52 weeks—versus about 30% for placebo (Bannowsky A et al. 2006).

Intrapenile injections can also be helpful. Six months of triweekly PGE1 injections for ED following bilateral nerve-sparing radical prostatectomy helped 67% of patients recover firm erections sufficient for sexual intercourse, compared to 20% for those who were not treated for their postsurgical ED (Carson CC et al. 2006). In cases of no response to PDE-5 inhibitors, combining them with intracorporeal injections could promote early return of natural erections (Raina R et al. 2006).

A study of pharmacological rehabilitation of erectile function following radical prostatectomy indicates that factors predicting failure include a rehabilitation delay of more than six months, no response to Viagra 12 months postsurgery, needing trimix injection doses exceeding 50 units, age over 60, and having more than one vascular comorbidity such as coronary arterial disease or hypertension (Mueller A et al. 2006).

In selected cases of ED after radical prostatectomy accompanied by low serum testosterone and not responding to PDE-5 inhibitors, testosterone replacement is successful. However, due to the risk of cancer flare-up, this therapy should be used with great caution and with close follow-up of the patient's serum PSA.

In some cases, when the neurovascular bundles cannot be preserved because of the cancer's extent or high malignancy, a penile prosthesis (see chapter 13) can be inserted during the prostatectomy or a few months later, with good results.

Treatment Acceptance, or Not

For his own peace of mind, a man with a sexual dysfunction should become an expert on his available treatment options and their possible results and remember that it is his choice to accept or decline any proposed treatment. Unfortunately, many men still refuse to discuss their sexual problems with their physicians. Several clinical studies have shown that despite the availability of simple, effective, safe treatments, fewer than 10% of men suffering from ED worldwide accept any treatment whatsoever for their condition. You may also be surprised to learn that about 50% to 90% of ED-afflicted men may refuse any further treatment beyond a first attempt or enter a treatment program but then simply drop out.

To elucidate motivations for seeking or refusing treatment for sexual dysfunction, Dr. R. Shabsigh conducted a unique study of "treatment-seeking behavior" in men aged 20–75 from six nations: the United States, the United Kingdom, Germany, France, Italy, and Spain. Of the 32,644 men screened with initial questionnaires, 2,141 men returned the follow-up questionnaires, which revealed some interesting findings. Regarding men who suspected they had ED, the United States had the highest proportion of men who sought medical evaluation for it, with a prevalence of 56%, compared to 48% in Spain and about 27% in Italy and Germany. The use of medications to treat ED was very low overall, ranging from 14% in the United States to 8% in France (Shabsigh R et al. 2004).

The most important incentives to seek treatment were the patient's self-motivation or pressure from his wife or sexual partner, and to a lesser extent, an article in the lay press, a television or radio show, or a TV, radio, or movie commercial. On the other hand, Shabsigh found that reasons for refusing treatment involved the false notion that ED is a normal consequence of aging, an expectation that it may resolve itself with time, being too embarrassed to

---

CRITERIA FOR CLINICAL STUDIES

For a clinical study to be considered unbiased and for its findings to be statistically significant and published in respected peer-reviewed journals, it has to fulfill some basic requirements: being randomized, prospective, placebo controlled, and double-blind. In lay terms, it must include a sufficient number of participants chosen objectively beforehand, compare the effects of the treatment of interest (in this case, a PDE-5 inhibitor) to those of a placebo (a "dummy pill"), and ensure total ignorance of the participants and researchers as to what is given to whom. In the course of the study, participants may be switched from one drug (or placebo) to another, with each used for a specified time and following a "wash-out" period.

The researchers take and record objective measurements and observations of the participants, and the participants may also answer questionnaires regarding the benefits and side effects they are experiencing. The results are computer analyzed for statistical significance in terms of the treatment's therapeutic effectiveness and safety compared to the placebo. The occurrence and severity of any side effects with the treatment (or placebo) should also be noted because side effects may prevent patients from adhering to a prescribed treatment regimen.

---

discuss it, or thinking that the problem did not occur frequently enough to merit therapy (Shabsigh R et al. 2004).

It is obvious that for many couples, the phenomenon of sexual intercourse transcends the simple ability to achieve and maintain a firm erection for a sufficient time for sexual gratification. It should involve intimacy and senti-mental, emotional, psychological, and romantic preparation for sex, with the active participation of the wife or sexual partner, in a relaxed and uninhibited atmosphere, according to each person's respective preferences.

What the majority of men with ED who are still willing to engage in sexual intercourse really want is to regain natural and spontaneous erections elicited by foreplay, and not by an artificial method that is required for every episode of intercourse and may entail unpleasant side effects. Those high standards could probably be met in the future with gene therapy (see chapter 11) or another means; those same high standards, however, may prevent millions of men in the present from using the treatments that are now available, even though these treatments could help them, albeit artificially, to develop firm erections and enjoy sex again.

Chapter Eleven

CONSERVATIVE TREATMENT OF ERECTILE DYSFUNCTION: ORAL AND TOPICAL MEDICATIONS

The curve is more powerful than the sword.

Mae West

Since the introduction of Viagra (sildenafil) by Pfizer, Cialis (tadalafil) by Lilly-ICOS, and Levitra (vardenafil) by Bayer-Glaxo, a marketing war has raged among their manufacturers. Those giant corporations spend an average of $400 million annually on advertisement and promotion of their products, with an eye on the huge international market and potential profit. In 2005, profits reached about $2.5 billion. Viagra currently holds about 60% of the world market, while Cialis and Levitra share the remaining 40%.

As a result, most people have heard about these phosphodiesterase type 5 (PDE-5) inhibitors, as they are the predominant drugs for erectile dysfunction (ED) in use and on the air, but know very little about them. Many people also have no idea that there are additional weapons in the anti-ED arsenal. This chapter covers the gamut of oral and topical drugs and other substances that offer patients different options in the conservative treatment of ED (Webster LJ et al. 2004, Frajese GV, Pozzi F 2005, Hatzimouratidis K, Hatzichristou DG 2005, Carson CC et al. 2004 & 2006).

PHOSPHODIESTERASE TYPE 5 (PDE-5) INHIBITORS

Full understanding of the PDE-5 inhibitors' mechanism of action requires a grasp of the salient features of erectile physiology. On sexual stimulation, nitric oxide (NO) is released from parasympathetic and nonadrenergic/noncholinergic nerve endings, and possibly from the endothelium of the blood vessels, in the penis. On entering the smooth muscle cells of the penile arteries and sinuses, NO stimulates the enzyme guanylate cyclase to convert guanosine triphosphate into cyclic guanosine monophosphate (cGMP), a potent smooth muscle relaxant and vasodilator. This in turn activates the enzyme called protein kinase G, the phosphorylation of other proteins, and the movement of calcium out of the cells.

That series of biochemical events relaxes the smooth muscles in the penile arteries and sinuses. The vessels' dilation enables blood to gush into the penis at high pressure, the sinuses' dilation occludes the penile veins by pushing them against the tunica albuginea, and the blood is trapped in the penis. The resulting erection is then made firmer by contraction of the muscles surrounding the penile shaft. Thus several pro-erectile substances play roles in producing and maintaining erection.

After a while, the antierectile enzyme PDE-5 spoils this happy event by breaking down cGMP into inactive GMP, leading to the gradual loss of the erection, despite NO's efforts to maintain it. During this struggle between pro- and antierectile substances is when the PDE-5 inhibitors intervene. These drugs block the action of PDE-5 on cGMP, thereby enhancing the smooth muscle relaxation of the arteries and sinuses and maintaining the erection. But remember that PDE-5 inhibitors do not have any effect on sexual desire, and they do not act in the absence of sexual stimulation.

Viagra, Cialis, and Levitra are all considered to be effective and safe (Carson CC, Lue TF 2005). The PDE-5 inhibitors share most of the same pharmacokinetics, that is, their activity and fate within the body over time, including their absorption, distribution, biotransformation, and excretion. (Certain pharmacokinetics particular to Cialis explain its longer period of action and its different side effect profile, as detailed later.) The characteristic speed, duration, effectiveness, and side effects for each PDE-5 inhibitor are important determinants in selecting the best medication for a man with ED.

Here are the facts about PDE-5 inhibitors as recently reported in the medical literature and presented at international meetings, which also complement my experience treating hundreds of patients with these medications.

Potency

For a PDE-5 inhibitor, potency is defined as the concentration of the drug that causes 50% inhibition of the PDE-5 enzyme and is measured as a value called the IC50.

	IC50 Range
Viagra	3.5–6.6
Cialis	0.94–0.99
Levitra	0.14–0.7

The smaller the IC50, the more potent the medication. As shown in the chart above, Levitra is biochemically the most potent. But frankly, nobody knows whether biochemical potency correlates with clinical potency and translates into higher efficacy in real-life use (Eardley I 2005).

Speed and Duration of Action

According to the advertisers, most men with ED would like to develop an erection as quickly as possible after taking a pro-erectile pill, without having to wait for one-half to one hour before being able to engage in sexual intercourse. What determines the speed of onset is the drug's period of bioavailability, which depends on the rapidity of its absorption into the circulation after being swallowed. The time in hours by which the drug reaches maximum blood-stream concentration is called Tmax.

	Tmax (hours)	Average onset (minutes)
Viagra (100 mg)	1–2	14
Cialis (20 mg)	2	16
Levitra (10 mg)	0.25–3	10

As shown in the chart above, these drugs' average times to onset of action generally correspond with their Tmax (Carson CC, Lue TF 2005). A recent comparative study demonstrated that achievement of a firm erection leading to successful intercourse occurred within 14 minutes in about 35% of patients given Viagra, within 16 minutes in 16% of patients given Cialis, and within 10 minutes in 21% of patients given Levitra (Wright PJ 2008). Food, especially a fatty meal, affected the absorption of Viagra and Levitra but not Cialis (see the following section for more about food and alcohol). In other studies, one-third of men taking Viagra developed an erection within 14 minutes and about 51% within 20 minutes, while onset of action for men taking Levitra was 14 minutes in 30% and 25 minutes in 53%. For Cialis, about 38% of the patients taking 10 mg and 52% taking 20 mg developed erections at or prior to 30 minutes, respectively (Jarrow JP et al. 2006).

In real life, the three compounds start acting within approximately 10–30 minutes after ingestion, with Levitra exhibiting the most rapid onset of action. Cialis and Levitra may start acting within 15–30 minutes. Viagra is usually taken about 30–60 minutes before intended sexual intercourse. However, a drug's rapidity of action may vary from one person to another and may also depend on several factors such as food or alcohol intake, degree of sexual stimulation, severity of ED, and the presence of anxiety or other emotional disturbances.

Conversely, the duration of a drug's action depends on its breakdown in the body. The time in hours by which the drug's concentration is reduced to 50%

of its maximal value is called T1/2. It takes about four or five half-lives for the drugs to leave the body completely.

T1/2 (hours)

Viagra (100 mg)	4–6
Cialis (20 mg)	17.5
Levitra (10 mg)	4–5

As the T1/2 for Cialis is much longer than for the other compounds, its duration of action may extend as well, to about 36 hours, far exceeding the four to eight hours' duration of the other two drugs—a potentially advantageous effect, and fully exploited in Cialis's ad campaign. A recent study revealed that about a third of ED patients attempted intercourse at least once within 12 to 36 hours after taking Cialis; this extension of a fixed schedule of intimacy provides a longer window of opportunity to enjoy more spontaneous sex (Shabsigh R et al. 2005b, Young JM et al. 2005).

Do Food and Alcohol Interfere with the PDE-5 Inhibitors?

According to several studies, eating a high-fat meal beforehand decreases the maximum blood plasma concentration of Viagra by about 30% and Levitra by about 18%, and the resulting decrease in Tmax delays the action of both drugs for approximately one hour. With Cialis, a fatty meal usually does not cause that delay because of the drug's prolonged duration of activity (up to 36 hours).

Alcohol, a well-known vasodilator, may affect the secretion of NO from the penile endothelial cells. In one study, moderate consumption (750 milliliters) of red wine one hour after taking Viagra did not cause any hypotension or other side effects (Leslie SJ et al. 2004). In another study, taking Levitra within four hours of consuming a moderate amount of alcohol not exceeding 0.5 grams per kilogram of body weight did not cause any side effects (Bayer-Glaxo Co. 2003). And in a third study, combining Cialis with moderate alcohol not exceeding 0.6 grams per kilogram of body weight did not produce any dizziness or marked drop in blood pressure. However, a significant drop in blood pressure did occur with Cialis when the amount of alcohol exceeded 0.7 grams per kilogram of body weight (about 180 milliliters of vodka; Carson CC, Lue TF 2005). Because the combined vasodilatory effect of alcohol and PDE-5 inhibitors may produce that result, the package labels for PDE-5 inhibitors warn against their co-administration (Wensing G et al. 2006).

Efficacy

Around 40 million men worldwide have been using PDE-5 inhibitors since Viagra's introduction, and few other drugs in the history of medicine have had so much psychological, social, and personal impact. Hundreds of international clinical studies (many, of course, sponsored by the manufacturers) involving thousands of patients have shown beyond the shadow of a doubt that Viagra, Cialis, and Levitra are equally and highly effective (and safe) for the long-term treatment of ED (Carson CC et al. 2004, Frajese GV, Pozzi F 2005).

Global success rates in enhancing sexual functioning range from about 42.5% to 80%, depending on the original cause(s) of the ED. With Viagra, for example, 42% of patients with ED after radical prostatectomy, 56% of patients with ED and diabetes, 70% with ED and hypertension, and 80% with ED after spinal cord injury experience improved erections (Carson CC, Lue TF 2005). Overall, by subjective or objective measures, in all age groups, and regardless of the severity and duration of ED, 70% to 80% of intercourse attempts with the use of PDE-5 inhibitors are successful, compared to about 20% to 35% with placebo. Even some patients whose ED does not respond well to intracorporeal injections of vasodilators (see chapter 12) can obtain a good response from treatment with PDE-5 inhibitors.

The success of the PDE-5 medications in helping men with ED develop and maintain good erections leads to significant improvement in their self-esteem, confidence, orgasmic function, sexual satisfaction, and sexual relationships but does not affect their libido (sexual desire). In most studies, PDE-5 inhibitors significantly improve scores on assessment tools such as the International Index of Erectile Function (IIEF) and the Sexual Encounter Profile for the majority of ED patients. Partner response and satisfaction is another important facet of these medications' efficacy; almost all studies reveal partner satisfaction with the results of PDE-5 treatment in about 75% of cases, compared to about 35% for placebo.

There is still some controversy regarding the beneficial effect of PDE-5 inhibitors for healthy men without ED. The reported results of increases in penile hardness and duration of erection before ejaculation as well as the decrease in the postorgasmic refractory period have not been fully proven in healthy young men. The few studies on this subject have included older men in their forties, who may have had risk factors that predisposed them to the development of ED. This may explain the apparent positive response to PDE-5 inhibitors.

Selectivity

The categorization "type 5" is meaningful in terms of the drugs' selectivity of action. The enzyme PDE-5 and 10 other types of phosphodiesterases, at different concentrations and with different structures and activities, exist in the penis as well as in various other bodily organs and tissues. Therefore the PDE-5 inhibitors block PDE-5 not only in the corpora cavernosa, but also in the vascular, digestive, and central nervous systems; tissues of the kidneys, bladder, urethra, heart, lungs, liver, and brain; blood platelets; and leg muscles. Viagra, Cialis, and Levitra exert different degrees of inhibition on some of the other phosphodiesterases as well, causing various side effects. For example, activity against PDE-6 in the retina can produce visual disturbances; activity against PDE-11 can produce muscle or back pain, although the precise cause of those symptoms is still obscure. Selectivity and associated side effects (see the following section) may play a role in the patient's choice of medication.

Side Effects, Drug Interactions, and Safety

Any man whose general medical condition prohibits sexual intercourse should not, under any circumstance, use any of these medications for sexual intercourse. Patients with severe cardiovascular disease (CVD; see later discussion), uncontrolled hypertension or hypotension, renal failure, or marked psychiatric disturbance should be included in that contraindicated group, unless cleared by the treating cardiologist, nephrologist, or psychiatrist.

Using a PDE-5 inhibitor is also definitively contraindicated in patients taking any types of nitrate, NO-donor medication, or the recreational drug called "poppers" (like amyl nitrate and butyl nitrate), as the combination can severely reduce blood pressure and may lead to dangerous, sometimes fatal complications. Other contraindications include a hereditary retinal lesion called retinitis pigmentosa, the use of certain alpha-blockers such as Cardura (doxazocin), and sudden loss of vision due to poor blood flow to the optic nerve. Severe kidney disease or marked liver dysfunction may necessitate medically supervised changes in PDE-5 inhibitor dosage.

Most of the side effects associated with PDE-5 inhibitors are shared by all three drugs. These side effects are typically dose-dependent, mild, transient, and abating with time and only necessitate discontinuation of the drug by about 3% of patients. Studies show that the most common side effects of PDE-5 inhibitors include headache, at an incidence of about 15% of patients using Viagra, Cialis, and Levitra versus about 3% with placebo; flushing of the face, at about 10% for Viagra and Levitra versus about 1% for placebo; and dyspepsia (indigestion with abdominal pains) after meals, at about 4% to 7% for the three drugs versus about 1% to 2% with placebo.

Less common side effects of PDE-5 inhibitors include nasal congestion and rhinitis (inflammation of the nose's mucous membranes), which occur in 4% to 9% of patients taking Viagra and Levitra versus 2% to 3% with placebo. Back and muscle pain occur mainly with Cialis, at an incidence of 4% to 10% versus 1% with placebo. Visual disturbances, such as a blue or green tinge, blurred vision, or oversensitivity to light, are most common among Viagra users, at an incidence of about 4%, and occur to a lesser extent with Levitra.

Sinusitis, diarrhea, and flulike symptoms occur in about 3% using Viagra and Levitra but not Cialis. Interaction with other medications is highest with Levitra (Carson CC, Lue TF 2005).

So far, no effect on spermatogenesis (sperm production) has been demonstrated with any of the three PDE-5 inhibitors.

Cardiovascular Risk Factors, Medications, and Complications

Spurred by recent epidemiologic studies confirming clear associations between cardiovascular risk factors, endothelial dysfunction, and ED, a group of cardiologists, urologists, and other experts from prominent medical centers convened the Second Princeton Consensus Conference to study the risks of sexual activity and adverse drug interactions with PDE-5 inhibitors for men who have, or may have, CVD. The group issued the following valuable recommendations about ED patients with CVD risk factors (Kostis JB et al. 2005):

> *Low-risk patients* can engage in sex and use PDE-5 inhibitors safely. This category includes people with fewer than three of these CVD risk factors: advanced age, male gender, smoking, hypertension, diabetes, high serum cholesterol and lipids, sedentary lifestyle, family history of coronary artery disease (CAD) at a young age, controlled hypertension, mild stable angina (anterior chest pains precipitated by effort or excitement and caused by ischemia (insufficient blood flow to the heart muscle)), successful coronary artery bypass surgery or revascularization with no residual ischemia or symptoms, mild valve disease, low-grade ventricular dysfunction, and being six to eight weeks or more after having had a myocardial infarction (MI, the death of a part of the heart muscle secondary to the occlusion of a major coronary artery normally supplying it with blood and oxygen).
>
> *Intermediate-risk or indeterminate-risk patients* require a full cardiac evaluation before they engage in sex. This category includes men with fewer than three of the following risk factors: moderate stable angina, having had an MI more than two weeks but less than six weeks ago, moderate left ventricular dysfunction or heart failure, and being prone to stroke or acute cardiac event because of clinically evident peripheral arterial disease.
>
> *High-risk patients* are those whose cardiovascular condition precludes engaging in sex until the condition is treated and stabilized. This category includes men with unstable or refractory angina, uncontrolled hypertension, severe congestive heart failure (CHF), high-risk arrhythmia (disturbance in the electric rhythm of the heart), having had an MI less than two weeks ago, noninflammatory disease of the heart muscle with obstruction and enlargement, and severe defect of the cardiac valves (especially stiffening or narrowing of the aortic valve).

The Consensus Conference further recommended that Levitra not be used concomitantly with antiarrhythmia drugs such as quinidine, procainamide, sotalol, or amiodarone. Furthermore, organic nitrates in all forms are strictly prohibited for use by patients taking any of the PDE-5 inhibitors; in emergencies when nitrates are medically necessary and other medications cannot be substituted, the patient should stop using Viagra or Levitra for at least 24 hours and Cialis for 48 hours before taking the nitrate.

Several well-controlled studies have confirmed that Viagra, Cialis, and Levitra have not directly caused any increase in the incidence of MI, any other major cardiovascular event, or death, except in cases of nitrate use or in patients with severe CVD with arrhythmia or cardiac failure (Mittleman MA et al. 2005). Although the PDE-5 inhibitors are considered safe and highly effective for men with minimal to moderate cardiac disease (Ravipati G et al. 2007), including patients taking multiple antihypertensive drugs, it is always best to refer men with high risk factors or any degree of CVD to a cardiologist for evaluation before prescribing a PDE-5 inhibitor or starting any other treatment for a sexual dysfunction. Because ED often indicates an underlying cardiovascular condition, close collaboration between the treating urologist and a cardiologist is greatly beneficial in a substantial number of cases.

Recent studies have demonstrated no significant effect of Cialis on resting coronary blood flow in patients with CAD, but compared to placebo, Cialis significantly increased myocardial blood flow in normal cardiac segments and especially in poorly perfused regions of the cardiac muscles (Weinsaft JW et al. 2006). Furthermore, PDE-5 inhibitors used in conjunction with prostaglandin inhibitors cause vasodilation of the pulmonary artery and reduce pulmonary arterial resistance and hypertension. They can also produce a mild decrease in blood pressure and an increase in the cardiac index and coronary blood flow in animals and humans (Schwarz ER et al. 2008).

Additional Drug Interactions

Drugs that should only be used with great caution by any men taking PDE-5 inhibitors include the alpha-blockers, such as alfuzocin, terazocin, doxazocin, and tamsulosin, used for the treatment of lower urinary tract symptoms (LUTS) secondary to benign prostatic hyperplasia (BPH). Their combination could cause a significant drop in blood pressure; an exception is the combination of Cialis with tamsulosin or alfuzocin, or taking Viagra in a 25-mg dose or less at an interval of at least four hours from taking the alpha-blocker. Other drugs like ketoconazole, erythromycin, and protease inhibitors (used for the treatment of AIDS) may interact with PDE-5 inhibitors and require dose adjustment.

Because the PDE-5 inhibitors and grapefruit are both metabolized by the same enzyme pathway in the liver, their ingestion together may cause major side effects and should be avoided.

Sudden Loss of Vision

Reports of sudden vision loss associated with each of the classic PDE-5 inhibitors prompted the U.S. Food and Drug Administration (FDA) to order the manufacturers to add warnings to the drug labels, although direct association of vision loss with the drugs is still unproven. Described as a form of stroke in the eye, with swelling of the optic disc, this condition is called nonarteritic anterior ischemic optic neuropathy, or NAION, and is characterized by painless loss of vision. It is apparently due to a vasoconstrictive effect (in this case, presumably of the PDE-5 inhibitor) on the artery supplying the optic nerve. Its estimated prevalence in the United States is about 1,500–6,000 cases per year.

NAION is more common in older men who have hypertension or cardiovascular problems, and some patients may be predisposed to it by a narrow angle at the port of entry of the vessels and optic nerves into the eye. NAION can also occur with the use of any PDE-5 inhibitor, even on the first dose. All patients taking one of these drugs should be advised of that possibility and instructed, in case of sudden decrease or loss of vision in one or both eyes, to stop taking the drug and seek immediate medical attention.

Over 43 cases of NAION associated with PDE-5 use for ED have been documented, and they share certain characteristics: patient age older than 50; low cup-to-disk ratio in the retina; history of hypertension, diabetes, heart disease, high cholesterol, and/or smoking; and history of eye problems. These similarities suggest that the actual cause of NAION may be those risk factors, rather than the drug. Patients with any of these risk factors for NAION should consult an ophthalmologist before using a PDE-5 inhibitor.

In a recent study of more than 44,800 patients who have used Viagra, the unadjusted incidence of NAION was 2.8 per 100,000 patient years, compared to 2.5–11.8 per 100,000 men (aged 50 or older) per year in the general public. This suggests that the incidence of NAION in people using Viagra is similar to its incidence in the general population not using Viagra (Sobel RE et al. 2006).

PDE-5 Inhibitors and Hearing Loss

Based on a case report from India of "a sudden bilateral profound and unremitting sensorineural deafness" in a 44-year-old man who had ingested sildenafil citrate (Viagra) 50 milligrams per day for 15 days (Mukhergee B, Shivakumar T 2007), the FDA found a total of 29 reports of sudden hearing loss associated with the use of PDE-5 inhibitors with or without accompanying ringing in the ears, vertigo, or dizziness. In most of the cases, as per the FDA news report issued October 18, 2007, the hearing loss involved one ear and was partial or complete, temporary in one-third of the cases and permanent in 70% of them.

Although no causal relationship was demonstrated between PDE-5 inhibitors, which were used by over 40 million men worldwide, and hearing loss, the FDA asked the manufacturers of Viagra, Cialis, and Levitra to revise product labeling and to display prominently the potential occurrence of such a complication with the use of any of the PDE-5 inhibitors.

Patients were advised to stop taking the drugs and to consult their physicians immediately if they experienced hearing problems.

Patient Preference

Exactly what attributes are men looking for in an ED treatment? In one study of this question (Eardley I et al. 2005), reliability of effect received the highest ranking (39%), followed by tolerability (31%), safety (26%), ability to concomitantly use other drugs (24%), low cost (22%), rapid onset (9%), and long duration of action (8%). Regarding the selection of a PDE-5 inhibitor, younger people may prefer the broader window of opportunity with Cialis, whereas older people may prefer Viagra or Levitra for their efficacy and reliability; these preferences, however, are not universal and may vary between different groups of men. In an another recent multicenter, randomized, open label, crossover European study comparing sildenafil and tadalafil preference for 291 impotent men, the most important characteristics for selecting tadalafil (71%) over sildenafil (21%) were erection hardness, time concern, better tolerability, intercourse satisfaction, choice of dosage, and number of successive intercourses (Eardley I et al. 2007).

Interestingly, the existing literature does not show a link between efficacy and patient preference for one PDE-5 inhibitor over another. Unfortunately, most of the many comparative studies that have been conducted worldwide (both independently and manufacturer supported) in an attempt to relate efficacy to patient preference with PDE-5 inhibitors suffer from significant design flaws that hinder proper interpretation of the data, and the results are often contradictory.

A recent study in Europe, sponsored by Cialis manufacturer Lilly-ICOS and comparing 20 milligrams of Cialis to placebo, demonstrated that about 63% of the participants attempted 25% of their sexual intercourses, and about 42% of the participants attempted about 50% of their sexual intercourses, more than four hours after taking the pill (medication or placebo). At least one attempt was made 8, 12, and 24 hours after taking Cialis (or placebo) by 87%, 75%, and 52% of the participants, respectively. The overall success rate for Cialis was more than 75%, versus 19% to 30% for placebo (Hatzichristou D et al. 2005). The study was meant to show that many men take advantage of Cialis's extended period of action (up to 36 hours), which theoretically provides more flexibility in timing sexual activity.

In comparative studies demonstrating a clear preference of the majority of patients for Cialis over its competitors, the major proposed reason for this preference is again its extended period of action, which can enable more spontaneity, more flexibility, and more so-called natural erections—that is, enough time for sex to arise more naturally without feelings of pressure to have intercourse on the medication's schedule—not affected by food or moderate alcohol intake.

The counterargument presented by Pfizer for Viagra and Bayer-Glaxo for Levitra is that the majority of men have intercourse within four hours from the time of planning it; their own manufacturer-sponsored studies show that over 80% of men proceed from planning sex and taking the medication to having sex within this time frame. Viagra's proponents also tout its long-term success rates, high efficacy, and safety over the past eight years in millions of patients worldwide, as well as its efficacy in ED secondary to spinal cord injury or antidepressant medication.

As for Levitra, biochemically the most potent of the three, its high efficacy, safety, reliability, and rapid action are the main arguments put forth for its preference, especially in one study that demonstrated a positive response to Levitra in about 30% to 46% of patients who failed on Viagra (Carson CC et al. 2006). Other studies, however, do not always confirm these findings; one demonstrated that Levitra salvaged only 12% of treatment failures in Viagra nonresponders (Brisson TE et al. 2006).

A review of the current literature reveals marked discrepancy regarding patient preference as well as evidence of biased research employing questionable methods and analyses to reach so-called definitive conclusions. I feel that it is impossible to compare Viagra, Levitra, and Cialis more objectively until head-to-head, independent trials fulfilling strict scientific criteria are conducted. The criteria (detailed in chapter 10) include complete independence of the manufacturers, randomized participant selection and group assignment, recorded etiology and baseline severity of ED, parallel group design with crossover of comparable doses of medication(s) and placebo for equal times, and strictly double-blind methodology. All participants should fill out questionnaires at the beginning of the study and after each treatment period within it (Eardley I 2005). The final analysis should also include assessment of partner satisfaction.

So which PDE-5 inhibitor is best? The candid answer to this million-dollar question is, we still do not know. Claims and counterclaims about specific advantages of the respective PDE-5 inhibitors are an ongoing debate. What conclusions can we reach? At present, I can only state that Viagra, Cialis, and Levitra are highly and equally effective in the management of

ED, with a global 70% success rate, regardless of the ED's causes and severity, and with an overall satisfaction for patient and partner of about 80%. Their successful use in impotent men may also improve their female partners' sexual function.

As far as the best PDE-5 inhibitor for any particular man with ED, that is an individual determination that depends on the medication's potency, efficacy, effectiveness, reliability, adverse reactions, and safety—and perhaps most important, the patient's expectations and preference. Because a PDE-5 inhibitor is intended to restore satisfactory erections, patients' reported outcome of treatment should be the gold standard by which to assess the efficacy of the drug. Therefore I encourage patients to try each of the three PDE-5 inhibitors and then stick to the one that suits them best. This method works well for the majority of my patients.

Patient Noncompliance

With the manufacturers' aggressive publicity and marketing of the PDE-5 inhibitors in the mass media, one would expect a rush of ED patients toward these drugs. Surprisingly, this is not always the case.

In an interesting study from Germany, in which 234 ED patients were treated with Viagra and followed for over a year, about 31% stopped taking the medication—despite its success. Why? Reasons included lack of opportunity or desire for sexual intercourse (in about 45% of the cases), lack of sexual interest on the part of the partner, cost of treatment, and occurrence of side effects (Klotz T et al. 2005).

Other reported reasons for noncompliance with pharmacotherapy include first dose unresponsiveness to the medication, the erection's artificiality and nonspontaneity, indifference of the partner to the man's sexual disturbance, fear of adverse reactions, poor sexual relationship, desire for a drug to target and cure the causes of the ED, and apprehension of possible medication failure during sexual intercourse.

Furthermore, among patients who initially respond successfully to a PDE-5 inhibitor, only about 45% continue the treatment after a period of three to four years. A recent review of the literature found that although about 40 million men with ED have been treated successfully with PDE-5 inhibitors, the treatment dropout rate is more than 50% worldwide. The presence of severe vascular disease, diabetes, and neurologic damage are associated with poor response to this mode of treatment (Hatzimouratidis K, Hatzichristou DG 2008).

Dropout reasons include poor follow-up results, fear of complications, co-morbidities (presence of other chronic disease), anxiety and/or depression, partner-related issues, limited sexual activity, loss of interest in these drugs and in sex, and especially the prohibitive cost of these medications, which is rarely covered by insurance companies and only partially covered (five pills) by Medicare. Some men may respond well to the PDE-5 inhibitors and yet may not be interested in pursuing the treatment anyway, especially if they are not sexually active or if they realize that restored sexual function is not as important to them as they had thought.

SEX IS MORE THAN AN ERECTION

Perhaps there is another reason for some patients' refusal of, or noncompliance with, PDE-5 inhibitors. This mystery may be illuminated by Meika Loe's book *The Rise of Viagra: How the Little Blue Pill Changed Sex in America*. According to Dr. Loe, "sex is a social business which involves two persons and not an individualistic process pursued by the male only. The success of Viagra is not due to a scientific breakthrough but rather a product of commercial interests with denial of the social nature of sex which was reduced to penile performance and degree of rigidity which determine a man's personal and social status" (Marshall Y 2004, 2776–2777).

To Dr. Loe and some other authors, Viagra represents a phenomenon called the "medicalizing of discontent," which is the "reinvention of sociopsychological problems as a simple medical condition" (Marshall Y 2004, 2776–2777). They suggest that ED was denuded of its psychosocial, emotional, and cultural aspects and reinvented as a simple physiological dysfunction to be cured by a drug—that "the problem was designed to fit the treatment, not the reverse" (Marshall Y 2004, 2776–2777), which may exacerbate the wider problem but still leads to increased sales and profits for the manufacturers.

Failure and Further Treatment

A failure with PDE-5 inhibitors may be due to such factors as the patient's age; the nature, etiology, and severity of his sexual dysfunction; improper use of the drug; gradual decrease in the response of the cavernous tissues to chronic use of the medication; a low serum testosterone level; or smoking, among other possibilities. One interesting study of nonresponders to Viagra found severe vascular lesions in the penis and atrophy of penile smooth muscle (Wespes E et al. 2005). And in a study of factors in success or failure with Viagra, response rates were best in cases of veno-occlusive disease and worst in cases of neurogenic ED, while age, smoking, and low IIEF score were the strongest predictors of poor response (Chia SJ et al. 2004).

An apparent treatment failure with one of these medications, however, is not necessarily the end of the story, as certain factors contributing to nonresponse may be discovered and corrected. For example, in cases when failure of a PDE-5 inhibitor may be related to low serum testosterone, testosterone replacement by gel or patches applied daily to the skin may result in a good response to the drug. For some patients with elevated levels of low-density lipoprotein (LDL, the "bad" cholesterol), treatment with a cholesterol-lowering drug such as Lipitor (atorvastain) can improve their response to a PDE-5 inhibitor. For other patients, a poor response to PDE-5 inhibitors may be due to low sexual desire, inadequate sexual stimulation, psychological disturbances, poor sexual skills, and/or conjugal problems, which should be addressed with psychotherapy and sex therapy.

An often overlooked, potentially reversible factor in failure with a PDE-5 inhibitor is inadequate patient instruction regarding the need to take four to six pills before giving up and to use the medications properly or risk a poor response. One study of 100 nonresponders to Viagra found that 45 did not use the highest recommended dose, 32 took it on a full stomach right after meals, 22 took it right before initiating intercourse, 12 ignored the fact that sexual stimulation is necessary for response, and 8 used the highest recommended dose despite medical contraindications. On follow-up, after proper instructions were given and reemphasized, 31 of those patients then responded to Viagra (Hatzichristou D et al. 2005). This highlights how important it is for patients to obtain—and follow—precise instructions regarding the use of the PDE-5 inhibitor medications.

Taking adequate doses of PDE-5 inhibitors, avoiding fatty meals for a few hours before and after their ingestion (particularly with Viagra and Levitra), and increasing sexual stimulation can salvage a substantial number of ED cases that did not initially respond to these medications. In certain cases, switching from one drug to another, such as trying Levitra with patients who are not responding to Viagra, may yield good results, although this practice is still controversial.

If treatment with these drugs is a definitive failure, the next move (with the patient's or couple's approval) is to try other nonaggressive therapies such as a vacuum device, intraurethral inserts, or intracorporeal injections (see chapter 12). Combining a PDE-5 inhibitor with inserts or injections may also yield good results, especially in cases of failure of these therapies alone (but the combination of PDE-5 inhibitors and intracorporeal injections is still not approved). A recent study involving patients with ED following radical prostatectomy, and for whom high-dose Viagra treatment had failed, combined administration of Viagra (50 milligrams) with four biweekly intra-penile injections of alprostadil (synthetic prostaglandin 1, or PGE1) for four weeks. This combination pharmacotherapy demonstrated good results on the patients' IIEF-domain scores, which reflect the degree of erectile improvement and the success of vaginal intromission and intercourse (Gutierrez P et al. 2005).

New Horizons in Treatment with PDE-5 Inhibitors

Confirmation of the following results by further studies, including my own, may open new horizons for the recovery of natural sexual potency in some ED patients:

> Long-term treatment with Cialis (20 milligrams) as needed for a period of three to six months (two tablets per week minimum) led to a 15.5% increase in peak systolic velocity through the penile cavernous arteries in men with normal vascular anatomy as well as in patients with inadequate blood flow. (Kocakok E et al. 2005, Sighinolfi MC et al. 2006)
>
> Long-term administration of PDE-5 inhibitors helps preserve smooth muscle function in the corpora cavernosa. (Hatzimouratidis K, Hatzichristou DG 2008, 128)

About 55% of patients who used PDE-5 inhibitors on a daily or every-other-day basis for several months recovered normal erectile function; most important, 95% of them maintained it even after stopping the medications (Sommer F, Schulze W 2005, Mirone V et al. 2005).

In view of these results, it is thought that the vasodilating effects of PDE-5 inhibitors may increase blood flow inside the penis during nocturnal erections, and that this increased oxygenation of the penile tissue may lead to its improved responsivity to neurologic (sexual) stimulation.

In addition to shedding light on the physiological action of PDE-5 inhibitors, other recent studies indicate further possible advantages of treatment with these drugs:

> PDE-5 inhibitors have been used successfully in the management of LUTS secondary to BPH (McVary KT et al. 2006); moreover, they also relieve the urinary symptoms and improve sexual function when combined with alpha-blockers.
>
> In patients with CHF and primary pulmonary hypertension, the combined use of Viagra and inhaled NO demonstrated a cardiovascular benefit of improved cardiac output due to their vasodilatory effect on the respiratory and systemic arteries. (Lepore JJ et al. 2005)
>
> PDE-5 inhibitors have yielded good results in the management of ED following renal transplant and pelvic surgery. (Zhang Y et al. 2005, Gallo L et al. 2005)
>
> Long-term treatment with Cialis improved endothelial function in men with increased cardiovascular risk by continuing to improve blood flow through the brachial artery (in the upper arm medial to the humerus bone) for as long as two weeks after Cialis's cessation, which may signify improved endothelial blood flow in the penis as well. (Rosano GM et al. 2005)

In the future, PDE-5 inhibitors may even find another wide use for the management of certain serious heart conditions (Hutter AM 2004). Furthermore, the success of these compounds in treating ED has boosted various research projects regarding cGMP and cAMP pathways in the bladder, prostate, urethra, ureter, and the female genital tissues, possibly opening new horizons in the pharmacotherapy of various genitourinary diseases (Uckert S 2008).

OTHER PHARMACOLOGICAL AGENTS USED FOR ERECTILE DYSFUNCTION

Both prior and subsequent to the discovery and widespread use of the PDE-5 inhibitors, several other oral and topical agents have been tried in the management of ED. These have not proven nearly as successful as the PDE-5 inhibitors but can be helpful in some cases and should be discussed with the treating urologist.

Apomorphine (Uprima)

A compound called apomorphine, which is unrelated to morphine but similar to dopamine, acts on the hypothalamus and perhaps the spinal cord's autonomic nuclei. It was introduced in 2001 for Parkinson's disease and ED, on the heels of the newly improved understanding of the positive effects of dopamine and other brain neurotransmitters on the physiology of erection. Apomorphine SL (a sublingual preparation) in 2- and 3-milligram doses was initially considered a breakthrough for ED treatment, as preliminary results of studies for FDA approval were very encouraging: a global success rate of about 65%, good tolerability, quick action within 10 minutes, and few minor side effects, including nausea, dizziness, yawning, and rare episodes of slow heartbeat and syncope (loss of consciousness) after the first dose.

Unfortunately, its subsequent use in larger studies over an extended time did not meet the initial high expectations, resulting in only a modest success rate of around 32% to 59%, and so far the drug is only approved for use outside the United States. Apomorphine could, however, be used concomitantly with PDE-5 inhibitors in certain cases when one or the other treatment has failed.

Trazodone

It was coincidentally observed, during clinical treatment for depression, that some patients taking the antidepressant Trazodone developed hard, sustained erections, some lasting for more than four hours. In a prospective, double-blind study at Boston University School of Medicine and Eastern Virginia Medical School, this drug significantly prolonged sleep-related erections, compared to placebo or other antidepressants. Additional studies demonstrated its successful experimental use as an intrapenile injection.

Trazodone's mode of action in erection is not well defined, although it is known to have an alpha-adrenergic blocking ability and to cause central inhibition of serotonin uptake in the brain. Peripherally, it appears to block the sympathetic system's constriction of the penile vasculature that would otherwise produce detumescence, and it may also have a central effect on the brain's sex centers that would prolong erectile duration.

Trazodone's peak action (on both depression and erection) usually occurs several hours after oral intake. So if the medication is taken in the evening, the best time for the patient to have intercourse will be the following morning, when the maximum effect may be experienced. The drug's side effects include drowsiness, sleepiness, dizziness, nausea, headache, insomnia, and lightheadedness in 10% to 20% of patients.

Unfortunately, additional clinical studies did not substantiate its initially promising results. With the introduction of the PDE-5 inhibitors, Trazodone's use for ED faded away and is now rare; the ED Guideline Panel of the American Urological Association does not recommend it.

Yohimbine and Herbs

Yohimbine, an extract of the bark of the yohimbe tree (*Rubaceae* and *Rauwolfia serpentina*) in Africa and India as well as the South American quebracho-blanco tree, has long been reputed to have aphrodisiac properties. In 1896, chemist Leopold Spiegel of Berlin was the first to chemically identify yohimbine and praise its action in increasing sexual desire and improving erectile function. Why and how yohimbine might work is still not fully understood, but as an alpha-2 ganglionic blocking agent, it blocks the constrictive effect of the sympathetic nervous system on the blood vessels, enhancing vessel dilation and facilitating increased blood flow to the penis.

Clinical tests of yohimbine began around 1970. Despite a few early reports of erections occurring in 25% to 30% of users (equivalent to the placebo effect in some large studies), and especially in those with psychogenic ED, recent controlled studies reveal no erectile benefit from yohimbine. There is no clear evidence of yohimbine's efficacy, except perhaps in some cases of psychogenic or mild organic ED and in cases of anorgasmia.

Yohimbine is generally safe if taken in the proper dosage under close medical supervision for no more than 10 weeks. Its maximum response (if any) may take two to three weeks or more to appear. Among its reported possible side effects is a rare central nervous system excitation, which includes elevated blood pressure and heart rate, increased motor activity, irritability, and tremor. Yohimbine may also cause headache, dizziness, nausea, insomnia, sweating, nervousness, water retention, lowered blood pressure, and skin flushing. Note that in patients with CVD or gastric or duodenal ulcer, yohimbine should only be used with caution. It should not be used by patients with severe or uncontrolled hypertension, except with extreme caution and under close medical supervision. Yohimbine is contraindicated for patients who are sensitive to it or who have severe kidney disease.

No true aphrodisiacs, herbal or otherwise, have been proven to exist, despite a recent claim from Italian researchers that nuts can significantly increase sexual desire. Some "rejuvenating" products or sexual stimulants such as Asian ginseng, L-arginine, and *Ginkgo biloba* might possibly increase sexual desire, facilitate penile microcirculation, and/or raise the penile concentration of NO, but there are no definitive studies of their effectiveness in treating ED. Other widely used herbs with anecdotal success include horny goat weed (several species of *Epimedium*) and a combination of fenugreek and ginseng. Randomized, controlled, double-blind studies are warranted to assess their efficacy and prevent their abuse for commercial gain. Meanwhile, I must raise a flag of caution regarding the use of herbal medicines for the treatment of sexual dysfunction (see the sidebar).

RISKS OF NONMEDICAL MANAGEMENT OF ERECTILE DYSFUNCTION

Several American studies have demonstrated that some so-called herbal compounds may appear efficacious in the treatment of erectile dysfunction because they also secretly contain Viagra. If such a drug is ingested without the man's knowledge, it may have serious adverse reactions with other medications he is taking (e.g., nitrates for cardiac disease), or he may be subject to serious medical complications (such as excessive bleeding during surgery).

On the topic of false advertising, let me also add a warning regarding claims in the mass media about the great value of "instructional videotapes" that supposedly help men overcome any sexual dysfunction and become "superpotent" lovers. Few of these videotapes are well prepared, professional, or helpful; most are no more than pornographic movies, with no genuine value in treating sexual dysfunction. They may, however, teach new sexual techniques to some inexperienced couples and relieve some of their inhibitions and ignorance about sex.

EXPERIMENTAL MEDICATIONS AND NEW FRONTIERS

Several new products are under experimental or clinical study. These include the following:

Another PDE-5 inhibitor, avanafil, from the U.S. manufacturer Vivus: taken orally; good preliminary results, with a rapid onset (within 15 minutes) and no effect of food and alcohol on its absorption and concentration

Calcitonin-based substances: taken orally; may assist in vascular dilation

Antiserotoninergic chemical agents: taken orally; may counteract the inhibitory effect of serotonin on the sex centers in the brain

The alpha melanocyte-stimulating hormone agonist melanotan, delequamine (has an action similar to yohimbine), oxytocin, calcium-channel openers, and naloxone: oral medications; encouraging preliminary results, but not much information yet regarding their mode(s) of action, rates of effectiveness, and adverse reactions

A newly discovered, as yet unnamed substance: undetermined mode of administration; increases the concentration of the smooth muscle relaxant cGMP, which plays a primary role in the development and maintenance of erection

Growth hormones: administered intramuscularly or intracorporeally; unknown action and results

Nitroglycerin and minoxidil: applied topically to the penile shaft or glans; may dilate the penile vessels and sinuses and increase blood flow to the corpora; in a few studies, results superior to placebo, but modest success and possible side effects

An ointment containing both PGE1 and the dermal permeation enhancer SEPA (standing for "soft enhancement of percutaneous absorption"): applied topically to the glans; very encouraging preliminary results with 1,732 ED patients, with a success rate of about 65% and only mild adverse reactions limited to the application site and subsiding within two hours (Padma-Nathan H, Yeager JL 2006)

Recombinant erythropoietin (a glycoprotein normally secreted by the kidney that stimulates the bone marrow to produce red blood cells): encouraging results in enhancing the regeneration of transected nerves in rats; could play an important role in the treatment of ED following radical prostatectomy

Neuromodulation and the use of neurotropic substances: following radical prostatectomy

A substance called PT-141: taken through an inhaler or by subcutaneous injection

Melanocyte-stimulating substance melanotan II, Rho-kinase inhibitor, and vascular endothelial growth factor (VEGF): administered either by intracorporeal injection or as part of gene therapy (see the following discussion); possibly acts on the brain sex centers or the penile vessels and sinuses to increase penile blood flow

Well-controlled, prospective, double-blind studies are warranted, of course, to assess the efficacy and safety of any potential ED treatment. Newly conceived methods like intraurethral instillation of NO, histamine, or cGMP are still in the experimental stage. Another, tissue engineering, has been used successfully in rabbits to replace severely fibrotic corporeal tissue with autologous cells cultured in the laboratory. The intact structural integrity demonstrated by the engineered tissue allowed normal copulation, ejaculation, and conception (Chen KL et al. 2006). If the preliminary results are clinically confirmed, this technique may find a major role in the replacement of severely fibrotic corpora subsequent to Peyronie's disease or infection.

The future treatment holding perhaps the most promise for permanent erectile restoration is gene therapy, by which various useful substances may be introduced into, and/or produced by, parts of the patient's own body. The penis, as an external organ that can be temporarily isolated from the general vascular circulation, is ideally suited to this approach. For ED, gene therapy entails intracorporeal injection of a specific DNA in one of several possible ways: through a plasmid vector (a self-replicating structure found in bacterial cells, which carries genes for various functions not essential for cell growth), an adenovirus or other nonvirulent virus, or naked DNA, which is considered the safest. The new DNA is incorporated into the nuclei of the target cells, where it is replicated, translated into messenger RNA, and ultimately transcribed into a specific product such as a protein.

That end-product of gene therapy for the cavernous tissues may help, for example, to improve NO's bioactivity and prolong a PDE-5 inhibitor's efficacy, thereby altering the intracavernous pressure on demand (Lau DH et al. 2008). Dr. Melman suggested that the presence of a defective NOS enzyme would increase the concentration of NO in the penile tissue or the H maxi-channel. By keeping the potassium channels open, this would prevent the influx of calcium into the smooth muscle cells and thereby dilate the penile vasculature (Melman A et al. 2008).

Gene therapy for ED has been conducted safely and efficiently in experimental trials with both animals and humans. At the 2006 annual meeting of the American Urological Association, Dr. Melman and his coauthors presented their results of the first human trial of "the transfer of a selective gene in the penis which can cause the production of endogenous proteins using the patient's own cells as bioreactors" (Melman A et al. 2006, 222). The nine patients in the study experienced no drug-related adverse reactions or abnormal laboratory findings, and the preliminary results in ED treatment were encouraging. Further controlled studies are warranted, however, with emphasis on efficacy and safety, before the wide application of this method.

A recently developed and most promising technique of gene therapy for ED uses the introduction of a double-strand suppressive RNA, called synthetic small interfering RNA, to downregulate the gene that controls the activity of the PDE-5 in the penis, thus inhibiting its negative effect and prolonging the action of the cGMP vasodilator. If further studies confirm the efficacy and safety of this method, it may open new horizons for the cure of some cases of ED.

Chapter Twelve

CONSERVATIVE TREATMENT OF ERECTILE DYSFUNCTION: VACUUM DEVICES, INTRAURETHRAL INSERTS, AND INTRACORPOREAL INJECTIONS

It's not the men in your life that counts, it's the life in your men.

Mae West

This chapter discusses three forms of conservative, nonsurgical, self-administered treatment for erectile dysfunction (ED) that can be utilized instead of, or in addition to, phosphodiesterase type 5 (PDE-5) inhibitors or other medications: vacuum pumps, intraurethral inserts of alprostadil (synthetic prostaglandin 1, or PGE1), and intrapenile injections of vasodilating substances into the corpora cavernosa.

Apprehension about injecting vasodilators directly into one's penis is one of the major reasons for refusing intracorporeal injections and for the high dropout rate associated with them. But interestingly, two-thirds of the participants in most clinical studies of patient preference choose the injections over a vacuum pump or intraurethral inserts. Compared to the other two methods, the injections can better reproduce a natural erection, with very high success rates, reaching about 70% to 85%; that reported range corroborates my personal experience with thousands of patients worldwide. Frequency of sexual intercourse is also found to be higher with injections than with a vacuum pump.

VACUUM PUMP THERAPY

The use of a suction device as an external erection aid is at least 75 years old but was not generally accepted by the medical profession until the mid-1980s.

Vacuum pump therapy is an effective, noninvasive technique that yields good results in a large percentage of men with ED, whether their dysfunction's etiology is organic, psychogenic, or mixed. It is especially helpful for men who can only achieve a soft erection. The use of a vacuum pump is mainly indicated for ED patients who are likely to experience drug-drug or drug-disease interactions if they were to take PDE-5 inhibitors, or for those who refuse other therapeutic methods.

Mode, Mechanism, and Method

The general mode of action of the vacuum pumps used as erectile aids is the creation of subatmospheric pressure around the penis. This induces the cavernous sinuses to fill with venous blood and the cavernous arteries and sinuses to dilate, resulting in their engorgement, increased blood flow into the penis, and subsequent erection (Broderick GA et al. 1992).

To initiate an erection, the man using one of these pumps prepositions a constriction ring (or a rubber band) onto the cylinder, into which he has placed his flaccid penis. He applies a generous amount of a lubricant jelly to the penile skin, the base of the penis, and around the rim, and to a few inches of the internal surface of the cylinder. He then uses the pump to create a vacuum of negative pressure around the penis.

It should, however, be emphasized that this method does not produce a completely natural erection, physiologically speaking, as it does not relax the intrapenile arteries or sinuses; these become engorged with blood because of the negative pressure around the penis, but the vessels do not directly dilate. So to maintain the rigid erection, the prepositioned constriction ring or band is slid off the cylinder onto the base of the penis, trapping the blood inside the penis. The man then presses the vacuum release button to remove his penis from the cylinder, and he is free to engage in sexual activity. Following intercourse, the constriction ring is removed and the erection subsides. Note that the constriction ring should stay in place for no more than 30 minutes, after which it must be removed. Keeping the ring in place for a longer period could result in severe damage to the penis.

Types of Pumps

Several types of vacuum pumps are available. Most consist of a plastic or silicone rubber cylinder with a pump attachment (see Figure 12.1).

Newer models have been streamlined into one basic component. A recently developed battery-operated model creates the vacuum with no active pumping on the part of the user. Other models are electrically operated by a touch button that simplifies the pumping process, especially for men with arthritis or neurologic diseases affecting the use of their hands.

Figure 12.1
Vacuum Erection Device

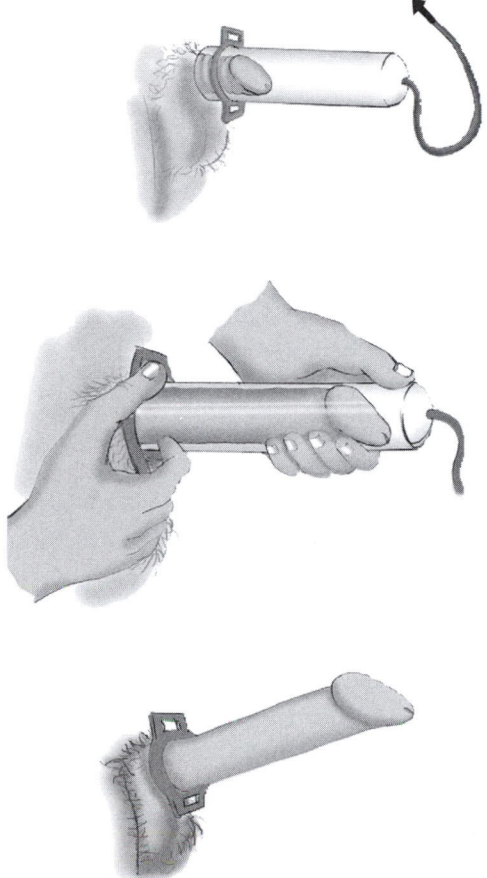

Courtesy of Alexander Balmaceda.

In one pump model, a soft constriction seal (rather than a hard ring) is pre-positioned between the base of the flaccid penis and the cylinder. It functions both as a vacuum seal for the cylinder, increasing the pump's efficiency, and as a blood flow–constricting device. Another model is constructed of semisoft, transparent silicone rubber shaped like a condom. After an erection is achieved by the pump's suction, the "condom" remains in place during intercourse. After intercourse, the vacuum lock is opened and the erection subsides.

Advantages

Although vacuum pumps do not produce every physiological aspect of an erection, they can help men develop firm erections sufficient for sexual intercourse.

These pumps do offer certain advantages such as simplicity of functioning, noninvasive character (as they are not surgically introduced into the body), and absence of systemic side effects, and they are relatively inexpensive. A particular advantage is that they do not preclude the return of spontaneous erections or the subsequent use of other forms of treatment. Vacuum pump therapy is a good alternative for ED patients who are not candidates for other forms of treatment.

The vacuum pump may also be used as an occasional change from intracorporeal injections, in addition to injections, in conjunction with a penile prosthesis to produce firmness of the glans penis, and sometimes even after the removal of such a prosthesis. Additionally, a pump can be used without the constricting ring as a means of so-called passive exercising for the intrapenile vessels by repeatedly filling them with blood. And in some cases of Peyronie's disease, a vacuum pump has been used to elongate the penis following surgical plaque excision and grafting.

Efficacy

Vacuum erection aids should certainly be part of the arsenal of any physician who treats male sexual dysfunction. All men with ED should have the opportunity to consider this form of treatment. Unfortunately, a lot of controversy exists in the medical literature regarding these devices. Some therapists claim excellent results after training and practice in a large number of patients; in some series, as many as 50% to 80% of users obtain satisfactory results, with about 50% to 90% of them achieving satisfactory erections at least once a week. Other studies, however, report such poor results and such high dropout rates that some sexologists have dropped vacuum pumps as a nonviable therapeutic option. Their overall success rate is about 55% over a two-year follow-up (Carson CC et al. 2006).

The bottom line is that vacuum pump therapy, when properly used, often works well to help the patient develop an adequate erection for sexual intercourse. Proper instruction and positive feedback are important for the pumps' successful use. It takes time to master, and a man who is interested in using a vacuum pump should not give up after the first try. The keys to its successful use are training, practice, persistence, and patience.

Patient Selection and Contraindications

In addition to persistence, successful use of a vacuum pump requires motivation, reasonable expectations, and approval and acceptance on the part of the patient and his sexual partner, along with manual dexterity. A thorough understanding of its mechanism of action, benefits, and limitations, and an acceptance of the possible side effects (see later discussion) are also essential for good results.

A man should never use one of these pumps without prior approval by his physician. In fact, all manufacturers require a doctor's prescription for purchase of a vacuum pump. Men vulnerable to priapism, and those with unstable cardiovascular systems for whom sexual intercourse may be dangerous, should not utilize this form of treatment. It is also contraindicated in men with severe penile vascular disease, bleeding tendencies, blood dyscrasia (any blood disease that causes bleeding, such as low platelet count or leukemia), or sickle cell trait or disease, and in men on anticoagulant therapy. Having any sores or ulcers on the penis precludes the use of a vacuum pump as long as the sores are present.

Safety, Side Effects, and Complications

Used as directed, vacuum pumps are safe, as long as the negative pressure generated does not exceed 200 millimeters of mercury (mmHg). They have few minor side effects, are not known to cause any significant complications, and may be discontinued at any time without after effects.

The patient should be prepared for a number of noticeable things that will happen to his penis during the use of the vacuum pump. Although the erection is unnatural, the penile length will probably match that of a natural erection, with a similar increase in circumference. However, because the constriction ring decreases subsequent blood flow into the penis, it will feel slightly cool. It may also look blue, and the veins will probably stand out because of the amount of blood trapped by the ring. Only the portion of the penis outward from the ring will be rigid, causing the penis to pivot and have a hinged appearance. Other disadvantages include penile pain and numbness, hemorrhagic spots on the skin, and cumbersome mode of use.

Depending on the type of constriction ring used, the man may or may not be able to eject his semen. Some rings block the urinary channel, trapping the semen until the ring is removed and the semen then drains out later in the urine (this causes no harm). Other possible effects include feeling an uncomfortable penile tightness and having a poor or absent orgasm because of discomfort and/or blocked ejaculation. There may be some superficial penile pain at first, but this goes away with practice.

Common problems in the use of vacuum pumps can be eliminated with proper education, experience, practice, hands-on training by an expert, and prompt correction of any mishandling or improper technique. Problems such as failure to obtain an erection, or to maintain it for more than a few minutes, may be due to an air leak resulting from poor sealing of the device to the skin at the base of the penis. This can be caused by a number of factors: inadequate lubrication, incorrect vacuum or ring size, excessive pubic hair, or a defect in the device itself. Using the proper size for the pump and the ring, applying a generous amount of lubricant at the base and over the shaft of the penis as well as at the end and over two inches inside the cylinder, and trimming the suprapubic hair are usually adequate corrective steps.

If pumping pulls the scrotal skin into the cylinder, it is helpful to remove any lubricant from the scrotum, properly angle the pump, use a smaller cylinder or ring, and pull the trapped skin out of the cylinder with a towel. Bruising and penile skin discoloration may be due to rapid or excessive pumping; pain during pumping may be due to a tight ring; and pain during intercourse or ejaculation may be caused by inadequate penile lubrication, prostate infection or inflammation, or lengthy sexual abstinence. Penile pivoting may be corrected by the development of a partial erection during foreplay, before the use of the vacuum pump. With practice and experience, most of these problems can be resolved to the couple's satisfaction.

INTRAURETHRAL ALPROSTADIL INSERTS

After the discovery that the mucous membrane lining the urethra is sufficiently permeable to absorb drugs, intraurethral inserts of alprostadil (PGE1) in the form of small pellets were introduced in 1995 as a relatively noninvasive therapy for ED. Although this treatment method has since declined in popularity among many urologists, it is still used in combination with oral PDE-5 inhibitors—and with a high success rate beyond 90%—for some men whose previous oral pharmacotherapy has failed. Intraurethral inserts may also be used to increase the rigidity of the glans penis in patients who have had a penile prosthesis implanted (see chapter 13).

Mode, Mechanism, and Method

When a pellet of 125–1,000 micrograms of alprostadil is inserted into the urethra, it is absorbed through the mucosa and diffuses into the corpora cavernosa, where it stimulates the enzyme adenyl cyclase to increase the production of a natural vasodilator in the smooth muscles of the penile arteries and sinuses. This substance, cyclic adenosine monophosphate (cAMP), by lowering the concentration of calcium inside the cells, causes vasodilation and increased blood flow into the penis. (About 90% of the inserted medication drains out through the veins and is inactivated in the lungs; only about 10% reaches the corpora to produce erection.)

Prior to intercourse, and after urination, the patient inserts a pellet into his urethra up to the collar on the applicator, which is called the medicated urethral system for erection, or MUSE. He presses the injector button to release the pellet inside the urethra, gently shakes the applicator to make sure that the pellet has dropped out, removes the applicator, and massages his penis for about 15 seconds (see Figure 12.2). For about 15 minutes after inserting

Figure 12.2
Intraurethral Inserts of Alprostadil (MUSE)

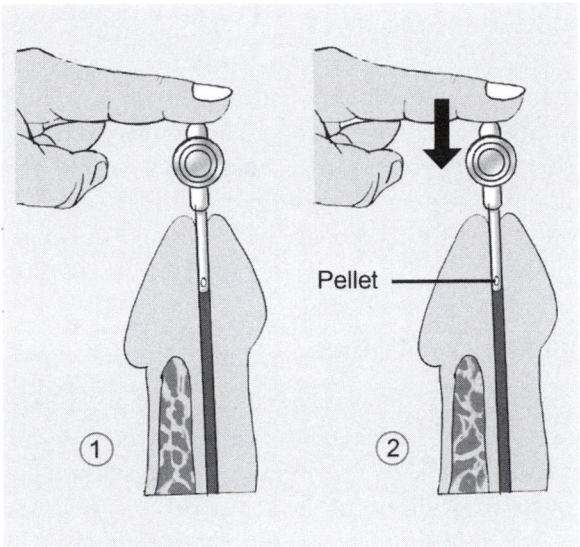

Courtesy of Alexander Balmaceda.

the pellet, he is to walk around or sit in a hot bath. He can then engage in sex once he develops a firm erection, which usually occurs within 15–30 minutes after the pellet's insertion.

Advantages, Disadvantages, and Efficacy

Advantages of treatment with intraurethral inserts include a natural type of erection within 5–10 minutes after insertion, without injection pain or any significant systemic side effects. Unlike intracorporeal injections, it does not produce prolonged erections, fibrosis, or penile curvature, even after long-term use. Its disadvantages, however, include poor long-term clinical results; a penile or urethral burning sensation in about 32% of cases; possible urethral bleeding and/or stricture, especially if the device is improperly used; the need for the patient to learn the technique and use the inserts properly; and difficulty of use by men who are extremely obese or lack manual dexterity.

Although the preliminary results of clinical studies in preparation for approval by the U.S. Food and Drug Administration (FDA) were very encouraging, with a reported success rate (especially in mild ED) of about 65%, subsequent reports on a larger scale and including all degrees of ED revealed much lower success rates of 35% to 45%, with less penile rigidity than with the intracorporeal injections.

Side Effects and Contraindications

Side effects of the intraurethral pellet are mild and include bleeding (from the urethra or in the urine), penile pain or burning, vaginal discomfort in the female partner, and dizziness. In about 6% of cases, a sudden drop of blood pressure with fainting may occur after the very first use, prompting some urologists to recommend performing the first insertion in the doctor's office with medical supervision. Note that this treatment method is contraindicated for intercourse without a condom with a pregnant woman because it may lead to high absorption of PGE1 through the vagina, with possible serious complications for the mother and possibly the fetus.

INTRACORPOREAL INJECTIONS

The main indications for this therapy include failure of PDE-5 inhibitors or intolerance or refusal of some men to use them or the vacuum device or the intraurethral inserts; ED with a severe psychological component; and ED following nerve-sparing radical prostatectomy with no response to PDE-5 inhibitors. Some 80% to 90% of patients for whom PDE-5 inhibitors fail may accept intracorporeal injection. Penile injections are also indicated for men who desire rapid onset of erection and persistent rigidity for an extended time.

The conditions most commonly requiring this form of treatment include arterial insufficiency, neurogenic ED, and mild to moderate venous incompetence. Selected men with psychogenic ED who failed or refused sex therapy and those with mixed vascular, neurogenic, or psychogenic ED are good candidates for injection therapy. The method seems ideally suited for a large number of men with organic ED, in selected cases of psychogenic ED, and especially for men with neurogenic ED or with mild vascular insufficiency. It is predictable, reliable, simple to use, aesthetically acceptable to the couple, reversible, and successful, and has few side effects.

The key to its success is producing total muscle relaxation in the penile vascular tissue. If a man with ED initially responds to injections in the doctor's office with good erections and has no aversion to penile self-injections, this therapy is a logical next step. However, because of its possible hazards and side effects, careful selection of candidates for this form of therapy is essential for optimal results.

INTRAPENILE INJECTION AS A TEST OF PENILE VASCULATURE

Obtaining a good erection from penile injection does not completely rule out vasculogenic problems, but it provides a good screening to indicate which patients may require more sophisticated vascular tests. For instance, if the patient develops a good erection within 15 minutes that lasts for more than 30 minutes, even after exercising, he may be considered not to have a severe penile venous leak. However, I must emphasize that this test may give false-negative and false-positive results and should not be used in patients who refuse intrapenile injection therapy.

Some nonresponders to the initial injection may respond to further injections of a combination of vasodilators, a higher dosage, or a more intimate setting. The test may also be positive in some patients whose moderate penile vascular disease can be overcome by the vasodilators. If it is positive, we can assume that no further vascular testing is necessary in about 70% of the cases. Although this test alone is not very accurate in definitively ruling out intrapenile vascular disease, it is extremely helpful in excluding the presence of a major venous leak; combined with duplex Doppler ultrasonography, it may diagnose penile arterial vascular disease.

Mode and Mechanism

Intracorporeal injections of vasodilators cause dilation of the penile arteries and vascular spaces or sinuses, as their smooth muscles relax under the influence of the drugs. With this arterial and sinusoidal dilation, there is a large inflow of blood into the cavernous tissue due to decreased resistance. The penile veins are then compressed against the firm wall of the penis by the dilated and engorged sinuses, decreasing the venous outflow to a minimum.

Within approximately 5–20 minutes—it varies from man to man—following intracorporeal injection of 2.5–60 micrograms of alprostadil or 0.25–1.00 milliliters of trimix (see the following discussion), a firm erection will develop that usually lasts 50–60 minutes or longer. Of course, the duration depends on the integrity of the penile vascular system, the type of drug(s) used, and the dose injected. However, psychological factors such as anxiety, fear, or stress may counteract the effect of the vasodilators by triggering the release of an increased level of vasoconstrictors into the blood. A patient should not exceed one injection every 24 hours or three injections per week.

The use of vasodilating substances over a prolonged period may result in a decline in the quality of the induced erections for some patients. On the other hand, some men report better spontaneous erections over time. This improvement in erection quality may be the result of a placebo effect, better compliance, increased elasticity, stretching, and dilation of the penile vessels and sinuses from their improved oxygenation, or increased sensitivity to the chemicals—or a combination of all these factors. There is no conclusive evidence on which to base an explanation.

Various Available Vasodilators

Papaverine was first injected with success by Dr. Virag in 1982, and the combination of papaverine and phentolamine was first used by Dr. Zorgnioti in 1985.

The current choices of intracorporeal injection ingredients are alprostadil alone, a mixture of papaverine and phentolamine (bimix), or a combination of alprostadil with papaverine and phentolamine (trimix), and sometimes with the addition of forskolin (quadrimix). My preference for the initial use of trimix, which is not shared by a significant number of urologists, who prefer to use injections of alprostadil alone, is related to a lesser degree of pain after injection, higher efficacy, longer action, and lower cost, albeit a higher incidence of priapism and penile fibrosis.

Alprostadil elevates the intracellular cyclic adenosine monophosphate (cAMP) in the vascular smooth muscles, resulting in their relaxation and in the vasodilation of the penile arteries and vascular sinuses. By inhibiting the enzyme phosphodiesterase, papaverine increases the concentration of cAMP and cGMP, resulting in prolonged smooth muscle and vascular relaxation and dilation of the cavernous arteries and sinuses. On the other hand, phentolamine or regitine is an alpha-adrenergic blocking agent, which counteracts the constrictive effect of the sympathetic nervous system on the penile vessels, resulting in their dilation and an increase in their blood flow.

Vasoactive intestinal peptide (VIP), a naturally occurring neurotransmitter, has also been used alone or with phentolamine. Preliminary results have not been very encouraging, as it is reported to have lengthened and widened the penis but not to cause firm rigidity. However, a report from Denmark on combined VIP and phentolamine indicated good results with few side effects (Gerstenberg TC et al. 1992). Ceritine, a mixture of six vasoactive compounds including 50% papaverine and 50% other vasodilators (ifenptodyl, atropine, yohimbine, piribedil, and dipyramidole), has reportedly been used successfully in France with few side effects. A study from Sweden reported successful intrapenile injections of nitric oxide (NO), with results comparable to PGE1, papaverine, and phentolamine, with very few side effects.

As yet, those compounds and their combination are not widely used and are not FDA approved. In the future, the use of NO alone (unfortunately, its action lasts only a few seconds) or one of its derivatives in cream or patches may become the treatment of choice. Other agents, such as VIP, calcitonin gene-related peptide, linsidomine, and sodium nitroprusside, are under investigation as injectable vasodilators but have not yet received FDA approval.

Types of Devices

An experimental pump system, implanted under the skin of the thighs or lower abdomen and connected to the corpora cavernosa, has been successfully used in the past to deliver the drugs intracorporeally, thus avoiding direct penile injection. Although this system was reported to result in better patient compliance and fewer penile complications, it has since gone into oblivion and is no longer used. An injection pen fitted with a small syringe, called Inject Ease and similar to that for insulin injection, has been successfully used and is reported to improve patient compliance and satisfaction. Another device, the Auto-Injector, injects the drug automatically from a prefilled syringe.

Proper Technique

If the patient, or preferably both he and his sexual partner, select penile injections after a full discussion of their hazards, risks, possible side effects, benefits, expected results, and all alternative modes of therapy, an acceptable dose is determined. Prefilled PGE1 injections of 10–20 micrograms, or a tri-mix formulation containing 10 micrograms or more of PGE1, 30 milligrams papaverine, and 1 milligram phentolamine per milliliter in a vial or prefilled syringes, is provided to the patient.

The success of this treatment depends greatly on properly educating and training the patient. Before dispensing medication and injection equipment, I make sure to demonstrate to the patient the normal anatomy of the penis and the proper site for the injection. I then explain techniques for handling the syringes or other injector in a sterile manner. A videotape or narrated slide presentation can also be very helpful. I then require him to self-administer the injections under my supervision at least twice before self-injecting at home. In addition, he receives an instruction sheet outlining the procedure. He is strictly directed not to exceed three or four injections per week and to call me immediately or go to the emergency room if any serious side effects, such as priapism, occur.

Some urologists provide unfilled syringes and a vial of trimix; others, citing safety reasons, provide syringes prefilled with the proper dosage instead of a vial. I leave the choice of prefilled syringes or other injectors to my patients. For those who are apprehensive, I recommend the Inject Ease; this usually eliminates needle phobia and increases patient compliance, and has decreased the dropout rate for injections in my practice. A follow-up appointment is scheduled for two to four weeks later.

These medications must be refrigerated and should not be kept at room temperature for more than a few hours. If the solution containing the vaso-dilators is properly refrigerated, its potency may last for six months or longer. Without refrigeration, its potency will only last for about two to four weeks. For men who travel extensively, a thermos bottle may be used to keep the solu-tion properly refrigerated, avoiding the excessive heat or cold that may affect its potency.

A consent form, carefully read, fully understood, approved, and signed by the patient, is mandatory before the administration of any injection. This con-sent form should emphasize the experimental nature of this procedure with trimix (which is still nonapproved by the FDA as a specific treatment of ED) and list all other treatment options, risks, potential hazards, and all known possible side effects of this therapy.

For the initial test injection in the clinic or doctor's office, low doses of vasodilators are used, especially in cases of psychogenic or neurogenic ED, to prevent overly prolonged erections. During this test, the patient is advised to stimulate his penis manually while watching an erotic movie, to better simulate the conditions and results he would experience at home after the injection. The combination of intrapenile injection and self-stimulation may cause an additive release of natural neurotransmitters and improves test erections in about 65% of patients.

Sample Injection Instruction Sheet

Instruction sheets vary from one physician to another, but for the protection of the patient and the doctor, an instruction sheet should always be given and reviewed. (I also provide instructions and training for use of an Inject Ease or Auto-Injector before dispensing these devices. The instructions I use—which the man takes home with him—are those provided by the manufacturer, with slight modifications.)

Safe Steps for Intracorporeal Injections

Make sure you fully understand the anatomy of the penis. If in doubt, please ask.
Handle vials, needles, and syringes in a sterile manner, as instructed.
Always discard the needle and syringe after use in a special disposal receptacle (available from a pharmacy or medical supply store).
Never reuse a needle or syringe.
Store medication-containing vials or syringes in the refrigerator.
Store all needles and syringes in a safe place, out of the reach of children.
Never inject at the same site repeatedly. Rotate your injection sites.
If you have any questions or need more information, please do not hesitate to call.

Procedure

1. Cleanse the injection site thoroughly with an alcohol pad.
2. Pull the cap off the needle while holding the syringe firmly with the other hand.
3. Retract the foreskin (if you are uncircumcised) and grasp the glans penis with the thumb and forefinger.
4. Stretch the penis and position it over the thigh.
5. Insert the needle up to its hub perpendicularly (at a 90 degree angle to the skin) at the injection site, at a clock face position between 1 and 3 o'clock or 9 and 11 o'clock (see Figure 12.3). Avoid any apparent blood vessels at the injection site.
6. Slowly inject all of the medication in the syringe by moving your thumb to the plunger and depressing it. (This movement is not necessary with the Auto-Injector.)
7. Remove the needle from the penis and apply pressure with the alcohol pad to the injection site for at least five minutes.

8. Clamp the thumb and forefinger of the other hand firmly at the base of the penis for approximately 30 seconds after the injection.
9. Massage the shaft of the penis gently.
10. Replace the cap on the needle. Discard the needle and syringe properly, as described above.
11. If, after the injection, you experience problems, such as dizziness, discoloration, or bruising of the penile shaft; absence of erection; or prolonged erection (lasting more than four hours), call us immediately or go to the emergency room.
12. If you do not achieve an erection following the injection, or in case of a weak erection, *do not reinject* before contacting us.

Advantages and Disadvantages

The advantages of intracorporeal injections include high efficacy with a success rate of about 85% (even in patients nonresponsive to Viagra); mimicking natural erection with a high level of spontaneity and discretion; and no

Figure 12.3
Intrapenile injections

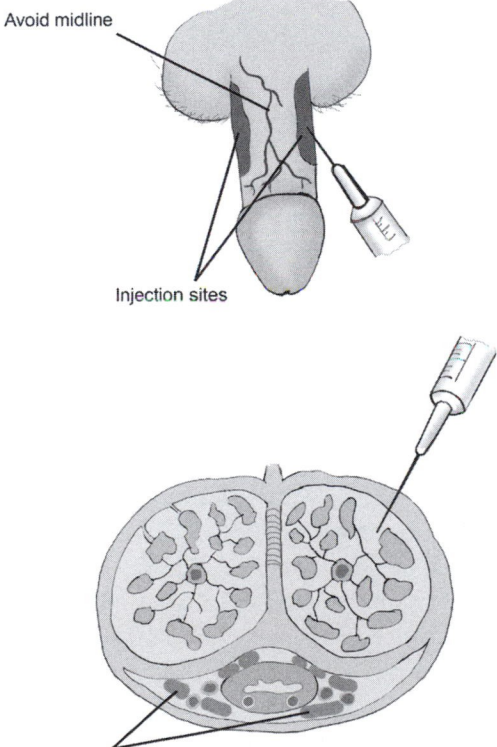

Courtesy of Alexander Balmaceda.

effect on penile sensations, ejaculation, or fertility (Carson CC et al. 2006). Optimal results, however, require proper training, periodic follow-up, and dose adjustment.

Among the disadvantages are pain at the injection site or during erection secondary to alprostadil (usually subsiding with flaccidity but may persist), priapism (prolonged erection lasting more than four hours), fibrotic plaques, hematomas, need for refrigeration, and lack of spontaneity. Others include the high dropout rate of about 40% to 60% after a few months and the need to master the injection technique, which can be difficult and cumbersome, particularly for men with extreme obesity or lack of manual dexterity. Furthermore, this mode of treatment may lead to dependence and usually does not relieve performance anxiety or improve the marital relationship. Its continuous use for years, if not covered by insurance, may be quite expensive (Althof SE et al. 1989, Hanash KA 1997, Lehman K et al. 1999).

Efficacy

According to recent studies and my own experience, PGE1 alone or low-dose trimix are probably the safest, most efficient vasodilators for penile injection. Trimix has none of the side effects of its constituents used individually in higher doses and can be effective even in cases of no response to the other drugs used alone. Each of the vasodilators in trimix acts on a different site in the vascular system of the corpus cavernosa; used together, they have a triple-header effect. Some comparative studies found similar efficacy, safety, and satisfaction with PGE1 and trimix, but more prolonged erections and a higher rate of priapism for trimix. Others, however, found better results, greater satisfaction, and fewer adverse reactions with trimix.

About 70% to 90% of men with ED for whom PDE-5 inhibitors failed and who have selected and used penile injection therapy were initially satisfied with the restoration of their natural erections, while 10% to 30% found it unsatisfactory. Its success depends on the root causes of the dysfunction, the age of the patient (diabetic men younger than 60 have much better results than older patients), type of drug, and dosage. Success also depends on the patient's compliance with instructions; cooperation with the physician; desire to improve; lack of fear, anxiety, or other psychological problems; and adequate sexual stimulation during foreplay after injection.

The overall success rate of penile injections depends on the makeup of any group to whom the injections are given. In a screened and carefully selected group, excluding all those for whom the injections are contraindicated, the success rate is about 70% to 90%. The satisfaction rate of the man and his sexual partner ranges from 50% to 78%.

Several studies confirm the claimed successful results of intrapenile injections of vasoactive drugs. One study from Albany Medical College of 141 patients treated with low doses of combined papaverine hydrochloride, phentolamine, and PGE1 found that after a follow-up of one year, 63% of the men were still using the injections, with a satisfaction rate of 89%. About 44% complained of occasional therapeutic failure, with at least one failed erection. Among those who stopped the injections, 31% did so because of a change in lifestyle as a result of surgery, divorce, or death of a spouse, and 25% because of diagnosed significant venous leakage or failed venous surgery. Only two participants recovered the capability for spontaneous erections (Bennett AH 1986). Several other past and current reports have demonstrated the high success rate and few side effects of these injections. A study from France on more than 800 cases followed over several years reported a success rate of about 90% with a low dropout rate (Virag R 1997).

Some men experience the return of spontaneous erections or notice a gradual decrease in response. Studies have reported the return of spontaneous erections in 8% to 30% of men using intrapenile injections. This may be attributed to psychological factors, such as overcoming performance anxiety, or to physical factors resulting from improved elasticity within the penile arteries and sinuses as a consequence of repeated dilation and improved oxygenation of the cavernous tissue.

Patient Selection and Contraindications

Psychological factors, difficulty in doing the injections away from home, and the sexual partner's refusal or negative attitude toward this form of treatment have a strong impact on a man's decision. Many men get tired of their dependence on injections, develop local or systemic complications, have difficulty mastering the technique, or lack any further interest in sex or in improving their potency. It has been noted that, in general, young men are more inclined to use these injections more frequently and for a longer time than older men.

A man selected for this therapy should be mentally stable, with no antisocial or aggressive schizophrenic behavior; well motivated; trustworthy; and willing and able to follow the physician's instructions. He should have no other medical condition contraindicating the use of intracorporeal injections of vasodilators. Contraindications to this form of therapy include uncontrolled elevation of blood pressure, severe diabetes, and severely diseased penile arteries. Also included are men who have sickle cell disease or trait, bleeding tendencies, unstable cardiovascular disease (CVD), angina, or cerebral ischemia. A man with chronic kidney failure; certain neurologic diseases such as parkinsonism, stroke, spinal cord injury, or tumor; mental disorder; marked hysteria; or low IQ would not be a good candidate for this therapy.

These injections may be dangerous for elderly men with marked CVD because of the possibility of a sudden drop in blood pressure and the development of arrhythmias (irregular heartbeats) that could precipitate an ischemic heart attack and possible death.

Other contraindications include patients who have severe venous leakage or liver disease, who have difficulty in mastering the injection technique, or who are unreliable and uncooperative in following the instructions. Patients who are overly concerned about the possible side effects of the injections, those on anticoagulants, and drug addicts are also poor candidates for this type of treatment. The use of anticoagulants does not constitute an absolute contraindication for the use of these injections, but it requires compression of the site of the injection for 5–10 minutes or more to stop any oozing.

Furthermore, patients with poor manual dexterity or poor vision are not good candidates for this form of therapy, unless their sexual partners are willing and able to learn the technique and perform the injections. Patients who develop side effects during the office test with the lowest test dose should be advised to consider other forms of therapy. Last but not least, extreme obesity may preclude the proper use of these injections, as the patient may have difficulty in retracting the fat pad covering his penis or in visualizing the injection site.

Psychological support is advocated prior to and during treatment. Penile injections may worsen the psychological disorders of patients with psychogenic ED, if proper counseling and sex therapy are not used concomitantly.

Safety, Side Effects, and Complications

With respect to the proper dose to be used at home, the patient's response to an initial dose should be assessed in the office. As an example, cases of psychogenic and neurogenic ED generally require a low dose of 2.5–5 micrograms of PGE1, whereas cases of severe arteriogenic ED generally require much higher doses, which could reach 30–40 micrograms of PGE1. All of these vasodilating injections are highly effective and usually safe, if properly used, with few minor side effects or adverse reactions.

One such reaction is priapism, a very prolonged, sometimes painful, nonerotic erection. It may occur in about 2% to 10% of patients using intracorporeal injections of PGE1 or trimix, depending on whether the strict criteria for patient selection and medication dosage have been properly applied. It is advisable for patients predisposed to priapism to use lower-dose injections of vasodilators. Such patients include those suffering from sickle cell anemia, thrombocytopenia (low platelet count), leukemia, polycythemia (increased red blood cells and elevated hemoglobin concentration), and multiple myeloma (bone marrow tumor with osteolytic metastases secondary to plasma cell dyscrasia). Men with psychogenic and neurogenic ED may experience a higher rate of priapism in general, up to 16%, particularly men with a positive response to a visual stimulation test of an erotic movie and a penile blood pressure index of more than 0.8. (See chapter 4 for more information on priapism.)

Other side effects associated with intracorporeal injections of PGE1 or trimix include development of localized penile fibrosis or fibrotic nodules inside the corpora, usually at the injection site, in 1.5% to 9% of cases, which occasionally produces penile angulation or Peyronie's disease if the patient persists in using the injections after the appearance of fibrotic plaques. These side effects occur especially with the long-term use of papaverine. There have also been reports of a sudden fall of blood pressure on standing, dizziness, headache, a metallic taste, pain from the injection outside the corpora or in the urethra, and cavernositis (infection of the corpora cavernosa). Some men experience penile swelling, penile paresthesia (abnormal touch sensations, such as tingling, burning, or prickling, in the absence of any external stimulus), decreased glandular sensation, penile angulation, and elevated liver enzyme levels (primarily with papaverine). Other rare complications include chronic pain and burning sensation in the penis, bruising at the site of injection with bluish-reddish discoloration, or a hematoma (collection of blood) under the penile skin.

PGE1 injections are associated with penile pain or burning after injection and during erection in about 20% to 60% of users, but other side effects are less common than with papaverine or phentolamine. The pain may be related to the acidity of the solution and may be relieved by adding sodium bicarbonate or the local anesthetic xylocaine to the injected solution. It has also been suggested that combining a lower dose of PGE1 with an increased concentration of phentolamine, or using bimix (papaverine and phentolamine) alone, may yield good results with less pain. The incidence of any adverse reaction is drastically reduced with the use of lower doses of trimix.

In a large-scale study comparing alprostadil versus bimix or trimix, the incidences of three side effects were as follows: (1) penile pain in 15% for PGE1, 1% for bimix, and 5% for trimix; (2) priapism in 1% for PGE1, 7% for bimix, and 10% for trimix; and (3) penile fibrosis in 1.7% for PGE1, 7% for bimix, and 7% for trimix (Lue TF 2004b, 43).

In general, the use of these medications is safe, with few serious complications, but appropriate patient selection and knowledge of contraindications are extremely important. There has been at least one reported death from an injection made inadvertently into the penile vein, which caused clotting of the blood in the vein and a pulmonary embolism (impaction of a dislodged clot in the lung's vascular bed).

The patient should receive periodic follow-up, with careful checking of the penis for any fibrosis and possible angulation or other side effects, the continuing efficacy of the injections, the occurrence of new medical conditions, the status of the cardiovascular system and blood pressure, and assessment of liver enzymes. The injections should be discontinued in case of side effects or complications.

Patient Noncompliance

If intracavernous injection is a simple, safe, and effective method to treat ED, why isn't it used routinely on all ED patients?

Some 10% to 20% of men with ED initially refuse this form of therapy, and about 20% to 60% discontinue it within one to two years. The reasons given most commonly by those who discontinued the injections included the artificial nature of the erections, dissatisfaction with the injections, recovery of spontaneous erections, high cost, insufficient rigidity for penetration, poor quality of response, reluctance to initiate lovemaking, concern about possible side effects, distaste for regular follow-up, and lack of spontaneity in achieving erections. Fear of needles, desire for a simpler method that does not involve their direct participation, and apprehension that the injections may fail at critical periods are among other significant reasons.

Recent studies with thousands of patients revealed high success rates of about 85%, but a significant dropout rate of 40% to 60% within the first or second year of treatment (De la Taille A et al. 1995; Fallon B 1995; Lehman K et al. 1999). It is usually quite difficult to predict accurately which patients will withdraw from intrapenile injections. Certain psychological factors, including low motivation, dissatisfaction with pharmacologically induced artificial erections, and persistent lack of self-esteem, may influence the discontinuation of this treatment. The first-year dropout rates of 20% to 50% identified by these studies confirm my own findings (Hanash KA 1997).

MEDICO-LEGAL ASPECTS OF TREATMENT WITH INTRAPENILE INJECTIONS

For a drug to be prescribed, it must be approved by the U.S. Food and Drug Administration (FDA), and then it can legally be prescribed for any use. Some drugs, however, have specific FDA-approved uses, meaning that the manufacturer petitioned the FDA for an approved-use designation, or official recognition that the drug is an effective treatment for a specifically named disease or condition. Without this approved-use designation, the manufacturer cannot advertise the drug as a treatment for that disease or condition.

Some manufacturers, in their medications' accompanying descriptive literature, include a statement to the effect that a drug is not intended to treat sexual dysfunction. This is a defensive move in case any problems develop. Some physicians still refuse to treat ED with intrapenile injections because ED is not on the FDA's approved-use list for injections of those drugs—even though PGE1 has been FDA approved for this use since 1998.

Much has been learned about injection therapy over the past few years, and it is now widely accepted as a safe and effective treatment. Although bimix and trimix are not specifically FDA approved for the management of ED, they can be used under certain provisions. Generally, the FDA considers the use of an approved drug for the treatment of an unapproved disorder to fall within the overall sphere of the "practice of medicine," which should be within the discretion of the treating physician. As a result of some past lawsuits, however, some physicians decide not to become involved in this type of pharmacotherapy.

Failure and Further Treatment

It has been shown that 6% to 30% of ED patients who try these injections fail to develop a good response to them. The most common medical causes are usually related to the vascular system, such as severe arterial disease or a venous leak, or commonly, a combination of arterial and venous disorders. Other causes may be improper injection technique, inadequate dosage, using only one drug (papaverine), psychological factors such as severe anxiety, or an inadequate level of endogenous vasodilators. Some of these failures could be salvaged with PDE-5 inhibitors.

As noted in chapter 11, some men who do not recover erectile ability with PDE-5 inhibitors or intrapenile injections alone may respond to a combination of the two. Combined treatment with intrapenile injections and PDE-5 inhibitors or vacuum devices may yield good results, especially for patients who develop a less than totally rigid erection with the injections. However, this combined treatment is still not officially accepted by the medical community or the FDA for fear of possible complications, particularly a sudden, severe drop in blood pressure.

Chapter Thirteen

SURGICAL TREATMENT OF ERECTILE DYSFUNCTION: PENILE PROSTHESES AND VASCULAR SURGERY

Everything will be okay at the end. If it's not okay, then it's not the end.

Anonymous

This chapter discusses the surgical treatments that may be appropriate in some cases of erectile dysfunction (ED).

If a patient is not a candidate for the conservative modes of treatment, if the conservative treatments fail, or if they are refused by the patient or his partner, the insertion of a penile prosthesis can be a viable option. Crucial factors in a thorough consideration of a prosthesis, before its selection and acceptance, include the mechanism of action of different types of devices, success rates, risks, benefits, possible surgical and postoperative complications, and cost.

As mentioned previously, certain men with ED may be candidates for vascular surgery to improve their penile circulation. An adequate penile blood supply is essential to achieve and maintain an erection, and insufficient arterial blood flow to the penis is a common cause of ED. But increasing the inflow may be only one part of correcting a penile vascular problem, as veins may leak or allow too much outflow for a man to maintain a rigid erection.

PENILE PROSTHESES

It is important to emphasize that a penile prosthesis does not cure the original cause of a man's ED. An implanted prosthesis mimics a natural erection by producing sufficient penile rigidity to enable penetration and thereby enjoy a satisfactory sexual relationship. Although the prosthesis itself does not improve libido, this restoration of erectile ability may increase sex drive for some men. Prostheses do not restore completely normal erections, nor do they restore any lost sensations, affect orgasm or ejaculation, or lengthen the penis (with a possible exception).

Although success and satisfaction rates for penile prostheses are fairly high, an implant is generally considered the treatment of last resort for ED, unless other modes of therapy are contraindicated or unsuccessful, or unless a prosthesis is selected by the completely informed patient himself. Almost all experts advocate trying all the noninvasive and least-invasive forms of treatment for ED before proceeding to the surgical insertion of a prosthesis. That progression makes good, logical medical sense. You do not want, as they say, to lock the horse out of the barn if there is another choice.

Patient Selection and Contraindications

Ethical and moral considerations should always complement the medical indications for any treatment. When a man requests a penile implant, specific indications apply. Following a thorough physical and psychological evaluation, the decision to proceed with the insertion of a penile prosthesis is made conjointly by the couple, the urologist, and, in cases of psychogenic ED, the psychologist or psychiatrist. But ultimately, the final decision on mode of treatment is up to the patient. If, after considering all options, risks, and benefits, he chooses a penile prosthesis, the doctor should—in most instances—respect his wishes, but only after thorough medical and psychological screening and counseling.

Proper patient selection is, again, the most important single factor in this treatment's success. A good candidate for a penile prosthesis is a thoroughly evaluated man whose ED has an irreversible organic cause that resists all other forms of treatment. The patient should not have any significant physical or mental impairment that precludes normal functioning of the prosthesis. Ideally, he should have appropriate motivation for the operation, a healthy desire for sex, and normal penile sensations and orgasm. His treatment expectations, and those of his sexual partner, should be reasonable and realistic, that is, a high likelihood of producing artificial erections with excellent rigidity for successful penetration and coital thrusting.

Successful manipulation of a penile implant (especially the inflatable type) also requires training, force and dexterity in the fingers, and full understanding of the device's function. Most patients can adapt, change some of their sexual habits, and accept an implant quite satisfactorily. For all the men with ED who wish to obtain and maintain a firm erection on demand, a penile prosthesis may seem like a good thing—but not all men with ED are good candidates for a prosthesis.

Men for whom the surgery would be risky, such as those with uncontrolled hypertension, severe cardiovascular disease, bleeding tendency, uncontrolled severe diabetes, or marked pulmonary disease, should be evaluated very carefully and cleared by the respective specialists beforehand. Prosthetic implantation is also contraindicated, at least temporarily, in the presence of any systemic, urinary, or cutaneous infections; those infections, when present, must be totally eradicated before surgery.

Men who have had strokes or other significant brain diseases, or who are partially paralyzed, may not benefit from a prosthesis. And in general, patients with psychogenic ED, psychosis, certain types of schizophrenia, acute or chronic depression, or personality disorders are not generally suited for a penile prosthesis.

The man whose ED is purely psychogenic could probably benefit instead from sex therapy, psychotherapy, oral pharmacotherapy, behavioral therapy, a vacuum device, intracorporeal injections, and/or intraurethral inserts. However, in certain conditions, when all the other approaches have failed and the patient is psychologically stable and properly motivated, a prosthesis may be offered after a thorough evaluation and the approval of the operation by a psychiatrist or psychologist. Postoperative psychological follow-up is essential for the success of surgery in these selected psychogenic cases.

The use of a penile prosthesis can help solve certain problems in a man's relationship with his sexual partner. But if the relationship problems stem from roots other than the man's physical inability to achieve and/or maintain an erection, then a prosthesis generally will not help, and behavioral sex therapy by a licensed counselor is the preferred treatment.

Selecting a Prosthesis

Choosing an appropriate prosthesis from the devices available should be a joint decision between the patient (or the couple) and the urologist. The main factors in selection are the patient's preference among the different types of prostheses; the respective advantages, disadvantages, success rates, complications, and average lifetime of specific devices; the surgeon's familiarity and success record with particular types of implants; and the cost. Large comparative studies have shown that the primary determinants of patient preference are cosmetic result, reliability, dependability, and reported satisfaction.

In most cases, the patient and his partner take part in a full discussion of these factors, review educational videos and charts, and have an opportunity to examine and manipulate samples of various prostheses before selecting the most suitable one. Possible complications associated with each type of implant, including infection, erosion, mechanical failure, and possible reoperation and removal of the prosthesis, are explained, as is the surgical procedure and the use of anesthesia. The expected results, based on reports of large groups of patients and on the treating urologist's personal experience, should be candidly presented. The couple is also informed of the position of the American Urological Association that there is no evidence that immunological (autoimmune) diseases, inadequacy, infertility, or birth defects occur in men implanted with an inflatable prosthesis.

The most important part of this meeting is that the patient and his partner are encouraged to ask questions. It is essential that they understand that a prosthesis produces an artificial erection that is usually not the full penile length that the man achieved naturally before his ED. It does not improve penile sensation, orgasm, or ejaculation. Its implantation is an invasive procedure that usually causes irreversible damage to the corporal tissue. The patient will, however, achieve an erection sufficient for penetration, allowing him to return to a healthy and satisfying sex life.

In my practice, I emphasize that this prosthetic implantation is elective surgery, not a matter of life and death. I also emphasize that following the insertion of the implant, antibiotic coverage is mandatory before any dental, surgical, or endoscopic procedures, to prevent infections of the prosthesis.

Medical and surgical considerations also influence the selection of a particular prosthesis. For example, paraplegic or quadriplegic patients who have poor penile sensation may benefit more from the insertion of a soft, inflatable prosthesis, which is associated with a lower incidence of skin erosion. On the other hand, a small, tight scrotum may not accommodate the pump reservoir of a two- or three-piece inflatable, or severe scarring from previous abdominal surgery may preclude proper placement of the reservoir in the lower abdomen for the three-piece prosthesis.

THE OPTIMAL LAST RESORT

In this new era of successful pharmacotherapy for erectile dysfunction (ED), selection of penile implants as the first line of treatment has dropped substantially, to approximately 5% to 10% of ED patients. About 70% to 80% of patients select one of the phosphodiesterase type 5 inhibitors (Viagra, Cialis, or Levitra) as their first choice. However, with increased public awareness of sexual dysfunction and a better education regarding its causes and modes of therapy, more men with ED are seeking medical advice and treatment. Furthermore, in cases of failure of all other conservative therapies, the insertion of a penile prosthesis becomes the next best option and can provide the patient with excellent results.

To some experts, a prosthesis is the most reliable and satisfying therapy for ED and the gold standard to which other treatment methods should be compared. To the majority of experts, however, a penile prosthesis is the treatment of last resort, despite its proven ability to produce an excellent erectionlike state, and should not be considered until all other ED treatment options have been tried and failed (or refused), or unless the patient's age and/or physical condition makes the other options infeasible. Whatever your opinion, the facts remain that penile prostheses are a means of treating ED indirectly without addressing its primary cause(s); each type has distinct advantages and disadvantages; they provide adequate, albeit artificial erections sufficient for intercourse; and when properly and successfully implanted, they do not negatively affect fertility or cause urinary difficulties. Although a prosthesis is not a panacea, it helps a man with ED achieve and sustain a rigid erection on demand.

Types of Prosthesis and Their Respective Pros and Cons

Since the introduction of the first inflatable penile prosthesis by Dr. B. Scott in 1973, more than 15 models, including semi-rigid, malleable, mechanical, and inflatable prostheses, have been marketed internationally and used on thousands of patients. Some of the original types have disappeared from use, and others have been improved. About 30,000–50,000 penile prosthetic implantations are performed annually worldwide. At present, two American manufacturers, namely, American Medical Systems (AMS) and Mentor Corporation, produce the majority of the penile implants most commonly used, including the malleables and the one-piece, two-piece, and three-piece inflatables.

Malleables

Some of the malleable implants are composed of pure silicone rubber. Others may contain an intertwined central metallic core or interlocking polysulfone rings coated with polytetrafluroethylene and connected by a spring-loaded cable, locking the rings into a column for an erection and unlocking them in the flaccid state. Still other models consist of a pair of silicone rods surrounding a core of silicone sponge, silver, or stainless steel. Implantation of these rods in the corpora cavernosa produces excellent rigidity, with the ability to bend the penis in the necessary directions. At present, the most commonly used malleable prostheses are the Mentor Acu-Form and the AMS 650. (Dacomed's Omniphase and Duraphase prostheses, previously widely used, are no longer available.)

After the insertion of a malleable implant, the patient has a constantly firm penis. This does not mean that he runs around with a noticeable erection all the time; the penis is always rigid, but it does not point upward, except when the patient himself bends it up for sexual intercourse. In a normal state, the penis with a malleable implant is bent downward toward the scrotum, where it should remain without flipping back upward (Figure 13.1).

Advantages of the malleables are their ability to be bent in different directions with good rigidity and flexibility, good results, low incidence of mechanical failure, simplicity of use, minor surgery involved in insertion (which can be performed under local anesthesia), low rate of postoperative complications, and low cost (about $950–$1,500 per pair of prostheses).

Figure 13.1
Malleable Prosthesis

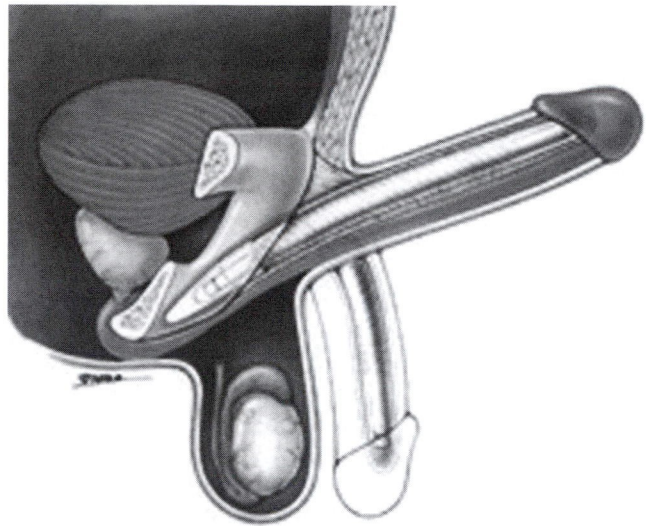

LGX™ Courtesy of American Medical Systems, Inc. Minnetonka, Minnesota. www. American Medical Systems.com.

Their disadvantages include permanent penile stiffness, lack of full flexibility and positioning, difficulty of total concealment, and possible buckling of the penis. Mechanical failure may occur with the breakage of the wire. Rigidity may be less than completely satisfactory, especially in men with long penises.

The couple satisfaction rate for the malleable prostheses has been reported to be quite high: over 90% in some groups of patients. This rate is similar to that with the inflatables. Older men, particularly, may find they prefer the malleable prostheses to the inflatable ones.

If a man with ED does not possess the mental or physical ability—for example, he lacks manual dexterity due to neurologic disease or arthritis affecting the hands—to operate an inflatable prosthesis, the insertion of a malleable prosthesis should be seriously considered. Another indication for a malleable implant is a case of Peyronie's disease (the "bent spike" deformity), resulting from severe and extensive penile fibrosis, in which it may be technically difficult to insert an inflatable device.

Inflatables

An inflatable penile prosthesis usually consists of two cylinders, a pump, and a reservoir that holds the fluid used to fill the cylinders. These parts are either incorporated into one device or are separate but interconnected and are placed inside the body. For all practical purposes, in the flaccid state, when the cylinders are deflated and contain only a small volume of fluid, the penis with an inflatable implant looks and feels quite natural.

The variety of inflatable penile prostheses available all share the same general hydraulic mechanism; that is, repeatedly squeezing the pump transfers fluid from the reservoir into the cylinders, leading to penile rigidity and erection at a 45 degree to 90 degree angle. This mimics, to some extent, the natural erectile process by which the heart pumps blood into the corpora in healthy men. After the completion of intercourse, the man squeezes the deflating valve or briefly bends the penis downward over a finger at midshaft, and the fluid drains from the cylinders back into the reservoir, causing the loss of erection.

The characteristics of each type of inflatable can be summarized as follows.

A one-piece inflatable is a pair of components inserted into the corpora cavernosa, each containing a cylinder, pump, and reservoir, all together in one piece. The term *one-piece inflatable* is actually misleading because it implies that the implant expands. In fact, with the one-piece inflatable, pumping simply transfers fluid from a rear-tip reservoir or an outer chamber to an inner nondistensible chamber, producing rigidity of the prosthesis without actually distending it. By repeatedly squeezing the end of the cylinder beneath the glans penis, fluid is transferred from the reservoir at the rear end of the prosthesis to the central cylinder, which becomes rigid, and full erection results.

Following intercourse, erection is terminated by bending the penis at midshaft to an approximately 45 degree angle for 15–20 seconds and compressing the cylinders. When the prosthesis is flaccid, fluid is held in the crural part of the cylinder and in the space between the outer silicone layer and the central Dacron sleeve. In the flaccid state, the one-piece inflatable is firmer than the multipiece inflatables, but still softer than the malleables. An advantage of the one-piece for obese patients is that it pulls the penis down from underneath the suprapubic fat pad, elongating the penis and giving it a more pleasing appearance in the flaccid state.

The one-piece inflatable may be the most difficult to manipulate of all the penile prostheses. Its operation is especially difficult for older patients with severe arthritis, neurologic diseases, or calloused and insufficiently sensitive fingers. After demonstrations by a physician or technician, the patient is usually able to function the prosthesis with a high degree of satisfaction, and his sexual partner may also assist with operating the device, if that is agreeable to the couple. The one-piece inflatable has been largely replaced by the other types and is rarely used nowadays.

Two-piece inflatables comprise a pair of cylinders in the corpora cavernosa, connected to a unified pump-reservoir in the scrotum above the testicles, just under the skin (Figure 13.2).

With the two-piece inflatable, squeezing the pump-reservoir repeatedly transfers its fluid to the cylinders, making them rigid. To release the erection,

Figure 13.2
Ambicor Two-piece Inflatable Prosthesis

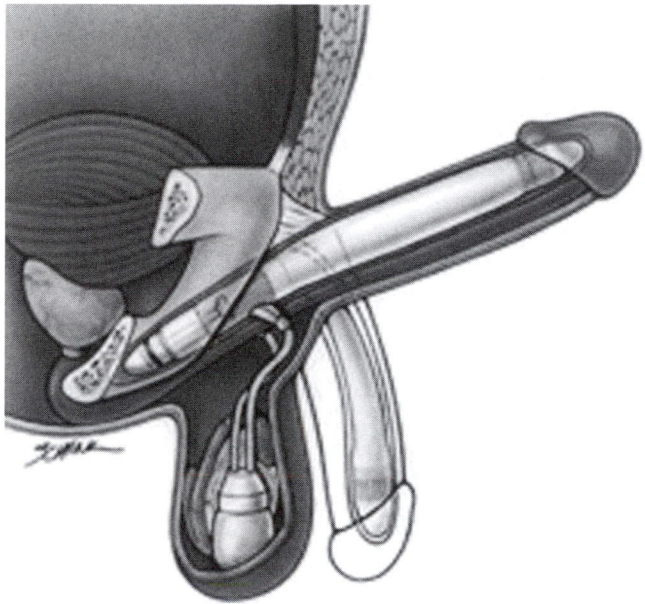

LGX™ Courtesy of American Medical Systems Inc., Minnetonka, Minnesota. www. American Medical Systems.com.

the man squeezes the deflation valve with one hand and compresses the shaft of the penis with the other hand, emptying the cylinders and forcing the fluid back into the pump-reservoir, or, in newer models, erection is terminated by bending the penis at midshaft downward over a finger and compressing the corpora for about 15 seconds.

Having a combined pump-reservoir implanted in the scrotum is a little like having a third testicle, but it is situated in such a way that no one would ever notice it unless the man pointed it out. It will take him a short time to become accustomed to it himself, and then he won't notice it either. Unlike the one-piece prosthesis, the cylinders in the two-piece inflatable do distend. During erection, the penis with a two-piece inflatable is less firm than with a one-piece but firmer than with a three-piece. The rather small volume of fluid contained in the system, about 15 milliliters, may lead to less than satisfactory erections for a patient who has a long penis.

Three-piece inflatables comprise a pair of cylinders in the corpora cavernosa, connected to a pump in the scrotum above the testicles, connected to a reservoir under the rectus muscles in the lower abdomen (Figure 13.3).

With the three-piece inflatable, squeezing the pump repeatedly draws fluid from the reservoir into the cylinders to produce an erection; squeezing the

Figure 13.3
Three-piece Inflatable Prosthesis

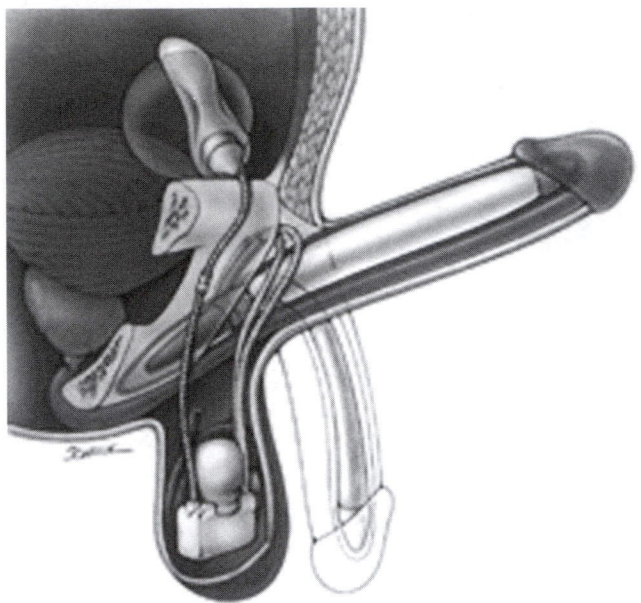

LGX™ Courtesy of American Medical Systems, Inc. Minnetonka, Minnesota. www. American Medical Systems.com.

deflation valve below the pump drains the fluid back into the reservoir to terminate the erection.

The three-piece inflatable may be considered the gold standard to which all current and future penile prostheses should be compared. The larger volume of fluid contained in this system, 65–100 milliliters, is enough to produce a hard erection. As a three-piece prosthesis is fully inflatable, it can possibly increase not only penile girth by 18–19 millimeters, but in the case of the Ultrex (see the following discussion), it can even increase penile length. These superior results are achieved for about $3,000 per total device.

In addition to number of separate components, the various models of inflatable penile prostheses also differ in materials, other design characteristics, and some particulars of function.

The most commonly used inflatable prostheses are from AMS: the three-component Ultrex (with length- and girth-expanding cylinders), 700 CX (girth-expanding cylinders), and 700 CXM (narrow cylinders); the two-component Ambicor; and the one-component Dynaflex. The AMS three-piece inflatables were originally composed of a single layer of silicone, which was prone to leakage and aneurysm formation. The cylinders' durability has since been improved by using triple silicone layers and a middle woven layer. A parylene inner and outer microcoating increases the lubricity of the silicone surface, thereby decreasing the wear from excessive friction. AMS also introduced an Inhibizone coating (with the antibiotics minocycline hydrochloride and rifampin) to prevent infection, and a silicone-ridged Tactile pump that transfers more fluid per squeeze and has a larger deflation site, providing for faster, easier inflation and deflation of the cylinders. A new three-piece inflatable prosthesis by AMS, called the LGX, has been advertised by the manufacturer of being able to increase the penile length by 2 centimeters and the girth from 11 to 18 millimeters (Figure 13.4). Clinical studies are warranted to confirm these claims.

Mentor's inflatables are constructed of polyurethane, with silicone polymer tubing and connectors and a silicone pump. All their implant components are now coated with a hydrophilic gel developed to prevent postoperative infection and also to provide lubrication by absorbing a great volume of water. Mentor also improved their Bioflex cylinders and the combined pump-reservoir, the Resipump, in their two-piece Excel, currently in clinical trials in the United States and available in some other countries. Mentor's three-piece inflatables include the Alpha 1, which features a Lock-Out valve reservoir to prevent spontaneous inflation or deflation, and the Titan, which is more lubricious than the Alpha models for easier implantation.

Compared to a malleable prosthesis, a one-piece, two-piece, or three-piece inflatable allows the man with ED to have more naturalistic erections, as they

Figure 13.4
CX, LGX deflated; CX inflated; and LGX inflated.

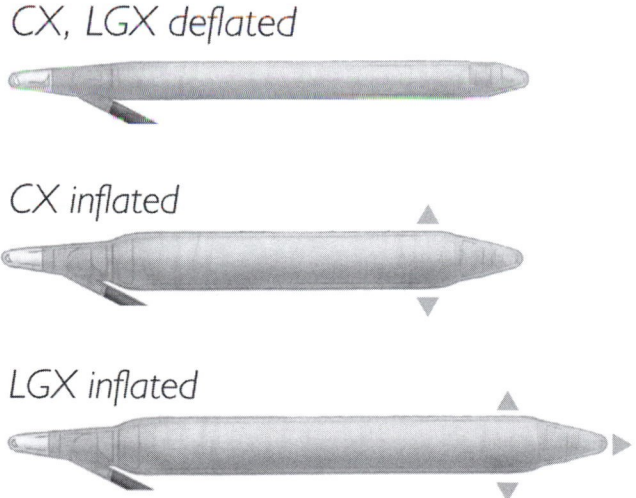

LGX™ Courtesy of American Medical Systems, Inc. Minnetonka, Minnesota www.American MedicalSystems.com.

occur only when he wants them and last for only as long as he desires. In addition to mimicking the normal erectile process, another major advantage is that the inflatables are totally concealable. An inflatable may also help to straighten the penis in cases of corporeal fibrosis and scarring, or in Peyronie's disease when no excision of the plaque is indicated and penile remodeling is a planned addition to the implant surgery.

The inflatable devices do, however, have certain disadvantages as well. They do not stiffen the glans (head of the penis), and the erections are not always as long or thick as the patient's normal erections used to be. With the one-piece inflatable, the low volume of fluid in the system produces an erection that is not as hard as with the two- or three-piece devices. Surgical insertion of an inflatable prosthesis, especially a two- or three-piece, is more difficult, takes longer, and usually requires hospitalization, general anesthesia, and longer postoperative care.

The complex hydraulic system also leads to a higher rate of mechanical failure than occurs with the malleables. Mechanical failure has been reported in approximately 3% of inflatables during the first postoperative year, 10% to 30% by five years, and 25% to 50% by 10 years, depending on the type of device. As reported in several large studies, the reliability of inflatables over five years of follow-up is 70% to 85%. A recent report from the Cleveland Clinic by Dr. Montague and associates on 380 patients who had undergone insertion of AMS 700 CX or CXM inflatable penile prostheses and been followed for a period of a median 91.5 months revealed a device failure in only 10%, with a 10-year Kaplan-Meier estimate of overall survival of the prosthesis of 74.9% and a mechanical survival of 81.3%.

When a penile prosthesis is removed because of mechanical or other complications and replaced with another implant, a particular type of inflatable, such as the AMS 700 CX or the Mentor Alpha 1, is usually selected at the urologist's discretion. After insertion of a new prosthesis, about 80% to 90% of patients are expected to have a functioning device for a period of five years. But the future is brighter and the rate of mechanical failure is steadily decreasing, thanks to new protective coatings, improved materials, and reinforced connecting tubes.

Preoperative Preparation and Treatment

Once a man with ED—having been educated as to the cause(s) of his dysfunction and the various therapies available to him—has opted for a penile prosthesis, the surgery must be carefully planned and the patient psychologically well prepared. The patient and his sexual partner (if he has one) must be fully informed of (1) the irreversibility of the surgery, which causes irreversible damage to the cavernous tissue and precludes the future use of any other forms of therapy for ED (except, of course, the insertion of another prosthesis);

(2) the artificial nature of the erections produced by a penile prosthesis; (3) the possibilities of a soft glans (when the cylinders do not reach the tip of the penis) and penile shortening; and (4) all the risks, hazards, and possible complications of the selected device. The patient and his partner are encouraged to ask any questions and to voice any concerns ahead of time. The surgeon, sometimes with the help of a psychologist or a psychiatrist, should assess the patient's and partner's expectations and attempt to identify all risk factors that could lead to an adverse outcome. Before proceeding with the implantation, I insist that the patient sign an informed consent form.

Treatment usually begins before the surgery as well. Preoperative treatment consists of therapeutic sessions and the assignments of at-home exercises to increase the couple's comfort in a variety of noncoital techniques and eliminate any performance anxiety or inhibitions. Other sexual exercises or training, such as for control of premature ejaculation (PE), are added as needed. The couple is instructed in effective communication, conflict resolution, listening skills, and elimination of negative thoughts that may inhibit arousal during sexual activity.

Preoperative management of any concerns or other psychological issues is also undertaken to prevent postoperative dissatisfaction or the worsening of any psychological or sexual problems (such as low libido or ejaculatory disturbance) associated with the ED. Marital conflicts are addressed to prevent their interference with the couple's sexual performance and compatibility. If the patient's partner has any sexual problems, or a negative attitude or misgivings toward a prosthesis, these must also be dealt with, to avoid a treatment failure, despite a surgical success.

If a man who has selected a penile prosthesis does not currently enjoy the companionship of a steady sexual partner, he receives training in the social and assertive skills that will enable him to approach a potential partner and start a sexual relationship without any anxiety, stress, or inhibitions about his ED and its treatment.

Postoperative Follow-Up and Treatment

After implantation surgery, the patient is likely to experience variable levels of discomfort, with possible penile and scrotal swelling. Moderate to marked discomfort may last four to six weeks. A brief or bandage is used to hold the penis up on the lower abdomen; if the prosthesis is an inflatable, it is kept fully or partially deflated. Intercourse and use of the prosthesis is not allowed for four to six weeks, and strenuous physical activities, such as heavy lifting, vigorous exercise, and jogging, are also prohibited.

During this postoperative period, the patient and his partner are sometimes advised to carry out Masters and Johnson's "sensate focus" exercises daily (Hanash

KA et al. 1994, 143). In postsurgical sessions with the treating therapist, significant issues, such as emotional reactions to the prosthesis, the appearance and size of the penis, and any anxieties about resuming sex, are discussed. The couple is encouraged to voice any concerns, uncertainties, or conflicts. Proper techniques for optimal use of the prosthesis are taught. Instructions are provided on different ways to initiate foreplay and sex and when to stop intercourse after ejaculation. How to monitor feelings of arousal and erotic sensations, rather than depending on erection to signal excitement, and how to proceed to intercourse under no pressure or demand are also discussed.

About four to six weeks following surgery, intercourse may be resumed, but without the inflation of the prosthesis. The man then meets again with the therapist, with or without his sexual partner, to evaluate overall satisfaction with the current sexual relationship, discuss any problems or difficulties that may have occurred in the resumption of intercourse, and help resolve any residual sexual difficulties or marital discord. The therapist checks the proper functioning of the prosthesis and ensures that the patient is able to operate it without difficulty.

Only then, if the patient is free of pain and infection, is he allowed to inflate the prosthesis for intercourse. At first, satisfaction may be low because of increased tenderness or decreased sensation, unfamiliarity with the mechanics, apprehension about malfunction, and/or a lack of natural sexual feeling. But with repeated attempts, satisfaction improves and the man and his partner soon adapt to the artificial erections. Using a lubricant is advised during the first several attempts.

A successful surgical result is not always synonymous with a successful sexual outcome. A man may not end up using his prosthesis for various reasons such as his partner's dissatisfaction with the results. After surgery, sexual issues other than the original ED can preclude adequate and pleasurable lovemaking; the patient may experience a low sex drive, PE, or difficulty in reaching orgasm, for example, or his partner's sexual dysfunction may prevent their full satisfaction. And a few men with ED simply want the prosthesis to boost their sense of virility and manhood, to feel that they are men again, without being particularly interested in resuming sex.

Postoperative follow-up is extremely important to ensure satisfaction with a prosthesis. Depending on any concomitant sexual issues, psychotherapy may be advisable and additional sexual homework exercises may be assigned. Some individuals or couples may require several follow-up postoperative therapy sessions to attain full sexual satisfaction.

Complications

As with all surgeries, there is a minimal risk of mortality and morbidity from anesthesia and implantation of a prosthesis. Intraoperative complications specific to penile prostheses are infrequent but possible. These include urethral injury, perforation of one or both of the corpora or the septum (the fibrous wall between the two), bleeding, hematoma, infection, and injury to the penile dorsal nerves and/or vessels. Extremely rarely, bladder or intestinal injury can occur during insertion of the reservoir for the three-piece inflatable prosthesis.

Postoperative infection and slight loss of penile length are infrequent but possible. Additional postoperative complications may be due to selection of a prosthesis that is too long or too short, or other technical or medical problems. Sometimes, pain can persist after implantation; penile sensation (especially in the glans) can decrease; the penis can buckle upward or downward; a component can erode through the corpora, urethra, scrotum, or skin; or the pressure of the reservoir on the penis, bladder, or intestines can lead to necrosis (tissue loss). Scarring can result in chordee (curvature of the glans and/or the shaft), asymmetrical positioning of the cylinders can result in deviation of the erect penis to one side, and cylinders not reaching the tips of the corpora can produce ventral curvature or so-called SST deformity of the glans (it looks like the nose of the Concorde airplane).

Prostheses are manufactured mechanical items; as such, problems may pop up, and breakdowns can be expected following their prolonged use. Eventual mechanical failure necessitating replacement of the device is also a possibility, amounting to about 10% over 10 years. In general, the more components in a prosthesis, the higher its chances of mechanical failure. A defective or broken implant requires revision surgery for its removal and replacement.

Postoperative psychological problems experienced by a dissatisfied patient or sexual partner are additional, potentially serious complications.

Infection

The most dreadful and disastrous complication with any type of prosthesis is infection. It may occur in 1% to 3% of virgin cases (during the first insertion), with this incidence increasing to about 5% to 18% during revision surgery. Infection is more common in diabetics (about 2% to 5%), especially if the diabetes is not well controlled; in immunosuppressed patients (up to 18%); and after single or multiple revisions in diabetic patients (8% to 18%). It also occurs more often in men with spinal cord injuries and chronic urinary tract infections, bedsores, or other systemic infections. It can have serious medical, medico-legal, and financial consequences, even—though rarely—including ischemia and destruction of penile tissue. It may take months, or even up to five years, before an infection becomes manifest.

The best treatment of infection is prevention, by using antibiotics before, during, and after surgery; using preoperative sitz baths with betadine solution; and shaving the genitalia in the operating room just prior to surgery.

Other preventive methods include careful preoperative preparation, proper tissue handling and strict sterile techniques during surgery, copious irrigation of the wound with antibiotic solution during surgery, and scrupulous postoperative care.

In the past, some urologists who used a surgical isolation bubble system to cover the site and prevent contamination reported a marked decrease in infection rate, but this technique is no longer in use. Recently, the AMS 700's new antibiotic Inhibizone coating and the Mentor Titan's hydrophilic coating (polyvinylpyrrolidone, which reduces bacterial adherence and absorbs the antibiotics in which the prostheses are immersed before and during surgery) have substantially decreased infection rates for patients receiving these inflatable prostheses to about 1%.

The classic management of an implant infection is to remove all the components, cure the infection, and insert a new prosthesis after several months. But because of severe scarring and/or fibrosis of the corpora following infection, surgery at that later date is technically more difficult, and the results are less likely to be satisfactory. For that reason, in selected cases of moderate infection without profuse purulent (pus) discharge or other signs of severe infection, some urologists prefer to remove the implant, treat the infection aggressively by irrigating the corpora with antibiotic and antiseptic solutions, and insert a new implant immediately or within three days. This salvage washout technique has been successful in over 80% of such cases (Brant MD et al. 1996). A modified version of the protocol, when used in surgical revision cases, reduced the postoperative infection rate from 11.06% to 2.86% (Henry GD et al. 2005).

Positive and Negative Outcomes

In a comparison of satisfaction rates among users of Viagra, intrapenile injections, and penile prostheses, the patients who underwent surgery reported significantly better erectile function and satisfaction than the patients who used the other therapies (Rajpurkar A, Dhabuwala CB 2003).

Success rates with penile prostheses vary. The original cause of the patient's ED may be a major determinant of this treatment's outcome. Men with diabetes-associated ED, for instance, have a higher success rate with these implants than patients who developed ED after surgery such as radical prostatectomy, or patients with ED subsequent to Peyronie's disease (for whom the overall success rate is high, about 75%). Other strongly influential factors in surgical—and sexual—outcome include patient selection, the surgeon's skills and experience, prosthesis type, presence or absence of marital conflicts and/or partner's sexual problems, penile length (flaccid and erect), loss of orgasm or ejaculation, and feelings of the patient and couple about the causes and treatments of the man's ED.

What Constitutes a Positive Outcome?

For implantation surgery to be considered completely successful, the surgical procedure as well as the postoperative recovery and treatment should be uneventful, without medical or surgical complications. No penile pain, discomfort, buckling, numbness, or paresthesia should persist more than a few weeks postoperatively; the flaccid penis should be easily concealable and natural looking, with no angulation; the patient should master the operation of the prosthesis; and the device should not malfunction (no spontaneous inflation or deflation) or fail.

Successful implantation also entails eventual complete satisfaction of the patient and his partner (if he has one) with the prosthesis. Satisfaction means good sexual, marital, and psychological adjustment, which may take up to a year after the surgery. The prosthesis should not produce psychological or marital problems in or between the partners; rather, it should meet reasonable expectations and lead to a fulfilling sex life, in which both people accept the prosthesis as a part of the patient's body; are satisfied with the length of the penis and with the rigidity, quality, and duration of erections; and are satisfied with the quality of sexual intercourse and can increase their frequency of intercourse at will. If, 6–12 months postoperatively, they "would do it all over again if they had to" without hesitation, this implies full satisfaction with the prosthesis.

Foundations of a Positive Outcome

Of the several medical and psychological factors that determine satisfaction rates with a penile prosthesis, the most important is how reasonable and realistic the couple's expectations are. Satisfaction also depends on the patient's personality and his own definition of a good result. Likely prerequisites for the combination of surgical success and full satisfaction for the implantee and his partner include the following:

Complete preoperative briefing regarding all the aspects of the prosthesis, what to expect from its use, and the proper selection of patients for its insertion
Maintenance of noncoital sex before insertion of the prosthesis
Free communication between the partners regarding sexual demands, frequency of sex, preferred sexual techniques, and skills in foreplay
Absence of psychological or marital problems
Understanding and acceptance of the physical changes that occur with age and with a prosthesis, which should not preclude fulfilling intercourse
Good psychological coping with the original ED and the couple's deep desire to contribute, along with the therapist, to its management and possible cure

The best way to handle any problem that may occur after prosthesis implantation is to anticipate the problem's occurrence and prevent it from interfering with a successful outcome. A team approach, in which several specialists in different fields conduct comprehensive education and discussion with both partners and treat any physical or psychological problems, is an extremely helpful preventive measure that may make the difference between satisfied and dissatisfied couples.

A therapeutic emphasis on the significance of foreplay and afterplay, adequate sexual stimulation, anxiety-free atmosphere, sexual fantasy, experimentation with different acceptable coital techniques, focusing on sexual sensations, and open discussions of fears and unrealistic expectations is of utmost importance. The treatment of associated conditions, such as PE, orgasmic disturbance, female sexual dysfunction and/or coital pain, marital conflicts, and other physical and psychological conditions, ensures a much higher satisfaction rate. Tenderness and affection in lovemaking, reaching orgasm by non-coital methods, choosing the right time and place, and avoiding making the sex act a performance test are additional important factors that can greatly benefit the couple.

Rates

Although the satisfaction rate with penile prostheses does not always match the surgical success rate—which may reach over 95%—it is nevertheless fairly high, at 60% to 90% or better. In general, men with a penile prosthesis are satisfied with the outcome and able to enjoy a fulfilling sex life. One study found the range of reported patient satisfaction with different types of inflatables was 60% to 92% (Brinkman MJ et al. 2005). In another, the inflatables were rated as "excellent" by about 79% to 98% of appropriately selected patients treated by experienced urologists, with a partner satisfaction rate of 75% to 96%. About 85% of patients with a penile prosthesis would advise this type of treatment to a friend, and about 75% would select it again if given a choice (Carson CC et al. 2006). Globally, partner satisfaction is about 60% to 85%.

Despite those generally high rates of success and satisfaction with penile prostheses, certain less than optimal reports have been collected from many implantees:

About 60% notice decreased penile length, thickness, and rigidity as compared to their erections pre-ED.

About 25% to 60% report decreased erotic sensitivity and orgasmic intensity. Implantees who do not achieve orgasm have decreased sexual desire and many other postoperative complaints such as penile pain, numbness, and prosthesis malfunction.

About 33% of implantees have sex less than twice a month; many implantees use their prosthesis quite infrequently because of physical, psychological, or marital reasons, and about 10% of diabetic implantees do not use their prosthesis at all.

About 10% to 20% of men do not use their prosthesis because of dissatisfaction with it. The partner is usually less satisfied with the prosthesis than the patient is; partner dissatisfaction, which is about 10% to 30%, may lead to severe marital or relationship problems if not prevented by discussion and/or counseling.

Dissatisfaction

Major reasons for dissatisfaction include unfulfilled or unrealistic expectations, decreased sexual desire, loss of sexual spontaneity, penile shortening, lessened orgasm, no real interest in sex on the part of one or both partners, marital problems, fear of injury, or a defective prosthesis. Other causes include partner dissatisfaction, penile pain during erection or intercourse, penile buckling, partner's vaginal or pelvic pain during intercourse, and anxiety or poor adaptation by the patient or partner to the presence of a foreign body in the penis.

The artificial nature of the erection, any malfunction of the prosthesis, dependency on an artificial tool, reduced size of the penis, failure to reach orgasm after surgery, decreased ejaculatory volume, and psychological problems may also contribute to dissatisfaction with the prosthesis. Another cause of dissatisfaction is when a man uses his prosthesis for intercourse without being sexually aroused; the act may be disappointing, as the man does not fully enjoy it and does not reach orgasm.

Believe it or not, many men simply do not realize that the majority of women are not very impressed by the size of the penis and are more interested in the tender, loving, romantic expression of sentiments during sex than in the sex act itself. The majority of men are erroneously convinced that their partners are looking for the kind of professional lovemaking portrayed in erotic or pornographic movies. These men may consider affectionate caressing and fondling, whispering of loving words, sentimental foreplay with sexual fantasies, and respect for the partner's sexual preferences to be an outmoded, ridiculous show of romanticism and a waste of time. Unfortunately, these men may not realize why their partners are not very interested in sex and why they fail to satisfy them despite their outstanding sex appeal or sexual abilities, which they assume have been further boosted by the prosthesis.

The artificial nature of prosthetic erections may lead to feelings that these erections and subsequent sexual activity do not result from the genuine desire and strong sexual arousal that reflect mutual physical attraction and affection. A partner may also feel increased sexual pressure from an ED patient who is now ready and able to have sex on demand. Sexual counseling and open, direct communication between the partners, encouraged and coordinated by a therapist, are highly recommended for couples experiencing these difficulties.

DISSATISFACTION DESPITE SURGICAL SUCCESS

Although the results as assessed by the surgeon may be entirely satisfactory, some men are dissatisfied with their penile prosthesis, mainly because of postoperative shortening of the penis, reduced sexual spontaneity, and unrealistic expectations. This disparity in perception can create tension between patient and physician.

A substantial number of lawsuits, the majority of them initiated by dissatisfied men, have been associated with this type of surgery. Some men complain that the doctor did not fully explain all of the details of the surgical procedure's medical and technical aspects, including all the possible complications (especially infections, which may necessitate the removal of the prosthesis) and the expected results. Some men claim that they did not understand the physician's medical jargon.

An excellent patient-physician relationship requires confidence and trust on the part of the patient and sound medical knowledge and expertise and caring on the part of the physician. The patient has a duty to satisfy himself by asking as many questions as he feels is necessary to obtain the in-depth information required to make an informed decision. He should seek a second (or third) opinion and refuse surgery until he is completely prepared to accept all of the possible results. The physician should use his or her expertise to provide the best possible care, recognizing his or her own limitations, and should be ready to refer the patient to a more experienced specialist, if necessary. He or she should patiently and thoroughly explain, demonstrate, and discuss all the various therapeutic options, with the risks, hazards, benefits, and possible complications of each, using layman's terms and spending as much time as the patient and his partner require. The physician and his or her team must also be available for postoperative care and counseling, including periodic follow-up.

VASCULAR SURGERY

As stressed in a consensus conference on ED held by the National Institutes of Health, "venous ligation and arterial revascularization procedures ... are incompletely standardized and validated techniques" (Lue T et al. 2004c, 39). In other words, these types of microsurgery are still not well defined and are not well accepted by many experts. They are complicated procedures that require a high degree of expertise, and their long-term results are usually not encouraging, except for carefully selected cases. For example, penile arterial revascularization is, at present, reserved for young men with ED caused by proven penile arterial occlusion secondary to a trauma, such as a fall on the perineum, and with no cardiovascular risk factors or history of smoking.

Revascularization of Penile Arteries and Veins

Several types of surgical procedures are used to achieve the goal of bringing more blood into the penis. By following proper diagnostic procedures, albeit with their possible pitfalls, the doctor may identify the arteries involved and the source of the blockage preventing adequate blood flow, for example, the aorta or one or more of its branches, especially the pudendal arteries that supply the penis. Bypassing or opening the blocked area may then be achieved by balloon dilation, laser, or other microsurgical techniques.

In cases of an occluded penile artery, blood flow to the corpora cavernosa can be surgically increased by selecting an appropriate source artery, routing it around the blockage, and connecting it to the penile dorsal or cavernous artery. This can be done by rerouting the source artery directly or by grafting the epigastric artery (under the rectus muscles in the lower abdomen) to the appropriate penile artery.

NEWSFLASH: PENILE ARTERIAL BYPASS

At the 2006 annual meeting of the American Urological Association, a study was presented of 80 men (aged 24 to 42) with erectile dysfunction caused by pure traumatic cavernosal artery insufficiency, as documented by duplex Doppler ultrasonography, cavernosometry, and pudendal arteriography. Between 1998 and 2005, the men underwent microvascular penile bypass surgery anastomosing the epigastric artery to the dorsal penile artery. Postoperatively, the patients exhibited marked improvement in their erectile process, penile rigidity, sexual satisfaction, and quality of life, with less psychological distress, less depression, and improved mood. Postoperative complications were mildly decreased penile sensation (in 21%) and penile shortening of about 1.09 inches on average (in 22%; Fantini GV et al. 2006).

It has been found that connecting a source artery to the dorsal penile vein may sometimes work even more effectively. This venous arterialization procedure reverses the blood flow in the selected vein so it works like an artery, resulting in retrograde increased flow into the corpora. A variation of this technique involves anastomosis of the epigastric artery to both the dorsal penile artery and vein.

A not yet proven procedure of balloon dilation, called penile angioplasty or penioplasty, is similar to ordinary coronary artery angioplasty, wherein a balloon is inserted into the obstructed vessel (in this case, the pudendal artery) to the point of the blockage and then inflated. The pressure exerted by the inflated balloon opens the artery by pressing the clogging material against the arterial walls.

The effectiveness of revascularization surgery depends on the individual and the specific cause(s) of the blockage, so what works for one man may not work as well for another. For example, venous arterialization with ligation (tying off) of the proximal and distal deep dorsal veins (see next section) is particularly successful in selected cases of vascular ED with atherosclerosis.

Reported short-term success rates of penile revascularization procedures range from 20% to 60%. The long-term success rate, beyond 5–10 years, varies according to whether success is judged subjectively (such as by patient report) or objectively (such as by arteriography), but does not exceed 25% in most studies. Furthermore, there may not be any correlation between the patency of the bypass (an open lumen with adequate blood flow) and its subjective or objective success (Kawanishi Y et al. 2004).

Various screening techniques (discussed in chapter 7) can identify those men for whom penile arterial correction is a viable option. A man's chances of being a good candidate improve if he meets the following criteria:

> He is relatively young (less than 50 years old).
> He is physically fit.
> He does not have any generalized vascular diseases.
> He has less than one or two additional risk factors (such as obesity and diabetes).
> He has a traumatic occlusion of the pudendal or common penile artery.
> He has a localized arterial obstructive lesion.
> He has normal veno-occlusive function.
> He is a nonsmoker.
> He has normal cholesterol levels.
> Color Doppler penile ultrasonography and pudendal arteriography confirm poor blood flow in the corpora and an obstructed penile artery.
> He is looking for a permanent cure for his ED by targeting the cause.
> He does not like the other options available, or they are unsuccessful or contraindicated for his condition, and he had no response to intrapenile injections.
> He fully understands and accepts the complexity and delicacy of the procedures; their relatively low success rates; and their risks, hazards, and possible complications.

Side effects of penile revascularization include hyperemia (engorgement and redness) of the glans, loss of sensations, edema (swelling) of the penis, shortening of the penis, and priapism.

Correction of Leakage

In men with primary ED who have never been able to achieve or sustain an erection, large veins may be leaking blood directly from the corpora cavernosa. Some men, particularly those with various medical conditions such as diabetes, Peyronie's disease, or hypertension, or with a history of trauma to the genitalia or of heavy smoking, may have diffuse (in more than one place) venous leakage, for example, from the corpora cavernosa to the deep dorsal penile vein, cavernosal or crural veins, or superficial venous system connected to the legs' saphenous veins. The leak is usually due to ineffective compression of the veins by the poorly dilated vascular sinuses during erection.

For ED caused by abnormal penile venous outflow, surgery may—or may not—be the answer. Dr. Tom Lue of the University of California at San Francisco elegantly classified different types of venous leakage according to etiology and advised therapeutic guidelines for each category, as follows (Lue TF, Tanagho EA 1987):

Type 1: congenital large leaking veins; a few of these cases may be treated by venous ligation.

Type 2: degeneration of the tunica albuginea enveloping the cavernous bodies, due to aging, Peyronie's disease, or other unknown factors; best treated with a penile prosthesis.

Type 3: direct injury to the sinusoidal smooth muscle, which precludes its full dilation and the consequent compression of the penile veins; treatment of choice is a penile prosthesis.

Type 4: inadequate or insufficient neurotransmitter release to produce arterial and sinusoidal dilation and their compression of the veins; best treated with intrapenile injections.

Type 5: venous shunt (abnormal flow of blood) between the corpora cavernosa and the corpus spongiosum; best treated with surgical ligation of the shunt.

Although these guidelines may be helpful in certain cases, they are not universally accepted or applied.

It has been found that most penile venous leaks stem from incomplete relaxation of the smooth muscles in the walls of the cavernous sinuses, with inadequate compression of the leaking veins. Mild cases can often be overcome by increasing arterial inflow and decreasing venous outflow. This can be accomplished with the use of a phosphodiesterase type 5 (PDE-5) inhibitor, perineal exercises, intracorporeal vasodilating injections, a vacuum pump, or a constricting ring placed at the base of the penis preparatory to intercourse. In severe cases, surgical ligation of the offending vein(s) is rarely successful because it does not address the leak's major cause or because the blood seems ultimately to find different channels for outflow after surgery.

For a localized leak, venous ligation, sometimes combined with dorsal vein arterialization to increase arterial inflow, may yield good results. For diffuse leakage, especially if combined with diffusely diseased intrapenile arteries, diabetes, and/or heavy smoking, insertion of a penile prosthesis is the treatment of choice. The initial enthusiasm for treating penile venous leaks by ligation gradually faded because of poor long-term results; most such cases are now managed with a constrictive ring or, preferably, with a penile prosthesis.

Accurate diagnosis of a venous leak and exclusion of coexisting penile arterial disease rely on Doppler ultrasonography, cavernosometry, and/or cavernosography (techniques detailed in chapter 7), which may also contribute to a successful surgical outcome. Proper patient selection, however, is the real key to success. A man is a good candidate for penile venous surgery or for embolization of the leaking veins if he is younger than 55; without severe generalized arterial disease; nondiabetic; with type 1 or type 5 venogenic ED; without severe penile arterial disease, as demonstrated by a good response to intrapenile injections; and a nonsmoker.

Although surgery would possibly work for some of the men excluded by the above criteria, their chances of success are much less. The association of venous surgery in borderline or poor candidates with overall poor results may explain the reluctance of the majority of urologists to perform it on most of their patients with this condition. Furthermore, although reported success rates after surgery were initially as high as about 60%, long-term follow-up for up to 10 years shows a drop to about 10% to 30% in most studies.

The reasons for failure include diseased cavernous smooth muscle, improper diagnosis, incomplete resection or ligation of all leaking veins, postoperative complications, presence of penile arterial disease or other etiologic factors, and formation of collateral veins (new venous channels forming off of the occluded veins) after surgery. However, as previously mentioned, venous ligation and revascularization are incompletely standardized and do not represent validated and accepted techniques for the management of veno-occlusive penile disease, except in rare, carefully selected cases. Insertion of penile prostheses may be considered the gold standard for most of these cases, especially if the other conservative modes of treatment have failed.

Several experts believe that the notion of venous leakage as the primary pathology in these cases of ED is inaccurate; rather, they attribute the generally poor results of ligation to a persistent pathology of the smooth muscles of the corpora cavernosa and to the performance of venous ligation on men whose ED is actually psychogenic and for whom the surgery may produce only a temporary placebo effect. Several studies have demonstrated a high success rate with the use of a constriction ring (without a vacuum pump) in the management of some of these cases instead.

A method called penile vein occlusive therapy (PVOT) consists of blocking the leaking penile vein(s) by injecting coils or sclerosing solutions (causing intentional scarring and occlusion) through the deep dorsal vein of the penis. The overall short-term cure rate with this technique was first reported to be about 52%. However, no long-term controlled studies of its efficacy were conducted, and PVOT has since faded away, except for anecdotal reports such as a recent study from Austria. In that study, 55 patients with veno-occlusive dysfunction and ED who did not respond to PDE-5 inhibitors were treated with venoablation of the leaking veins with a sclerosing solution, aetoxysclerol 3%. The procedure resulted in a 63.6% success rate and no serious complications; 35 patients were able to develop firm erections sufficient for vaginal intromission without additional therapy (Herwig R et al. 2006).

Chapter Fourteen

TREATMENT OF PSYCHOGENIC ERECTILE DYSFUNCTION

The content of a man's character is not where he stands in times of comfort and convenience, but where he stands at times of challenge and controversy.

Martin Luther King Jr.

In the past, the majority of cases of erectile dysfunction (ED) were attributed to psychogenic factors, and ED patients were generally referred to psychiatrists or psychologists for evaluation and treatment—typically with poor results. Nowadays, purely psychogenic ED accounts for only about 15% to 25% of all cases, but psychosocial factors may combine with organic causes in an additional 45% of men suffering from ED (Lue T et al. 2004a). Psychosexual therapy alone or in conjunction with medical treatment, especially with a phosphodiesterase type 5 (PDE-5) inhibitor, is the preferred approach for both psychogenic and mixed psychogenic/organic ED.

SEX THERAPY AND PSYCHOTHERAPY

Therapy for ED should be provided by a team consisting of a urologist, an expert psychologist or psychiatrist, and, if needed for the couple, a marriage counselor—especially if the patient has significant psychological, psychosocial, interpersonal, and marital problems, or if he has failed or refused medical treatment, or if his partner has significant sexual or psychiatric disturbances. Basic education of the couple regarding normal sexual functioning and the causes of their sexual disturbance(s) is the cornerstone of a successful therapeutic plan.

Psychotherapy may be useful as an adjunct to medical therapy with PDE-5 inhibitors (Viagra, Cialis, or Levitra) and may be helpful in certain cases when pharmacological treatment has failed because of psychogenic factors contributing to the dysfunction. The major goals of sex therapy and psychotherapy for ED are reduction of performance anxiety, focus on sensual pleasure, enhancement of the man's self-confidence and self-esteem, elimination of taboos and misconceptions about sex, improvement of sexual skills and communication between the partners, and modification of negative sexual attitudes and thoughts.

Sensate Focus

The pioneering 1970s work of Masters and Johnson, with subsequent modifications, remains the foundation of sex therapy. It involves eliminating performance anxiety, fear, embarrassment, guilt, and lack of confidence in one's sexual ability. It encourages the discovery of additional sensual regions in the male and female body and teaches the couple to focus on sensual awareness and pleasurable sensations during sexual arousal, without obsessing over the quality of erection or the so-called successful outcome of intercourse.

Masters and Johnson's sensate focus technique, adopted by many sex therapists worldwide, is a program focusing on a gradual increase in sexual stimulation and satisfaction, with minimal performance demands. The couple is given sex homework to be carried out two or three times per week for three to four weeks, during which time they are also to refrain from any sexual intercourse. They are instructed, meanwhile, to continue with mutual sexual stimulation by first exploring and discovering their nongenital pleasure spots, before gradually moving to the sex organs, providing each other maximal pleasure but without any type of penetration. Additionally, using educational and behavioral methods, the therapist encourages and teaches sexual and nonsexual forms of sensual communication.

Then, once the couple feels relaxed, able to communicate freely with nondemand forms of stimulation and mutual pleasuring, strongly motivated, and confident, they may resume intercourse. The man, who may have previously been so obsessed with the quality of his erection that he was distracted into becoming a spectator during sex, is encouraged to reassume the role of an active participant. He is also encouraged to regain his self-esteem and full confidence in his sexual abilities, without the inhibitions or anxieties that, by decreasing his focus on arousal, disrupt proper sexual functioning.

Anxiety and Depression, and Their Management

Traditional approaches to psychogenic ED, based on Masters and Johnson's work, concentrate on anxiety reduction, desensitization procedures, cognitive-behavioral intervention, relationship counseling, and education about sexual stimulation techniques (Rosen RC 2001). In certain situations, especially if sex therapy fails, medical treatment with a PDE-5 inhibitor is added to these tools of psychological management, often with good results. Nowadays, many clinicians even prefer to treat their patients with PDE-5 inhibitors alone, without resorting to sex therapy, unless pharmacological management fails.

Sexually related anxiety is considered the most common pathway leading to sexual dysfunction (Masters WH, Johnson VE 1970), but other psychiatric conditions may also contribute to ED's etiology. One such disorder is depression, which may be linked with severe affective (mood) and sexual disturbances in a bidirectional way. There is a high prevalence of depressive symptoms in men with ED, although the direction of causality is often debated; that is, does depression cause ED, or does the sexual inadequacy itself cause the depression? Treatment of severe depression by a psychiatrist may involve psychotherapy, antidepressants, and even electroshock therapy. Ironically, using certain antidepressants can exacerbate sexual dysfunction.

Minor depression, on the other hand, may only require the correction of maladaptive interactions between the patient and his environment. He may be able to accomplish this by the use of relaxation exercises, positive and constructive thinking, the application of certain rules, and the adoption of realistic goals and expectations in life. Examples of the actions in this approach include the following:

Learning to be more assertive, optimistic, extroverted, and involved in social activities

Practicing doing things that he likes

Rewarding himself with personal gifts such as nice clothing, a pleasurable vacation, or a coveted vehicle

Working on regaining his self-esteem and self-respect in general, and his confidence in his sexual abilities in particular

Wearing rose-colored glasses to ward off being disturbed by minor daily incidents

Being bold enough to take calculated risks and aware enough to enjoy every moment of happiness

Being willing to try to enjoy his sexual experiences without hang-ups, anxiety, fear, or inhibition

Working on Relationship Issues

Marital or relationship discord, which is so commonly associated with sexual dysfunction as either a cause or effect, may require the help of a counselor if the couple is unable to resolve it themselves. Certain behavioral changes, however, can work wonders if the couple is ready to implement them (Hanash KA et al. 1994):

Bringing back the romance in the relationship: stirring up the ashes to revive the flame of physical and emotional attraction; going back to the courting days to use their romanticism, sweet words, and simple gestures of respect and affection

Focusing on developing a mature love: characterized by loyalty; caring; sharing; companionship; friendliness; and a relaxed, fulfilled sex life

Respecting differences: resolving conflicts through positive dialogue, while avoiding insults, derogatory and sarcastic remarks, and bitter arguments

Accepting the partner's faults and virtues: encouraging and reinforcing positive behaviors and minimizing criticism; not expecting him or her to change character and beliefs overnight

Opening the inner world to the partner: sharing fears, hopes, insecurities, emotions, and needs; communicating in a gentle and respectful way, without inhibition or shame; allowing the chance to know each other in depth, thereby making the relationship stronger and more mature

Maintaining interest in the partner as an ever growing and changing person: sharing sorrows and joys, successes and failures

Avoiding blaming the partner: confronting problems maturely and courageously, taking personal responsibility for actions

The need for complete relaxation and avoidance of any stress during the sexual act, with total acceptance of the partner as an active member of the couple with all due respect

Learning how to practice sex, which may require years of training, not only to learn the proper techniques, but more important, to acquire the ability to listen to your emotions and express them during the sexual act; this would definitely improve the quality of any sexual performance

To learn how to experience sensual sensations through mutual caressing; fondling and massaging the erogenic spots all over the body, besides the genitalia; and focusing on the exciting sensations provided by each spot

To communicate freely and without any shame or embarrassment regarding the reciprocal preferred techniques of sexual stimulation and the aversive ones

To let the body react naturally to the sexual sensations, without any inhibition or attempt to control them

To apply a personal rhythm for sexual expression, without trying to emulate some applied standards

To learn how to breath deeply and relax completely during the sexual act

Intimacy, romanticism, compliments, and affection are important ingredients for optimal sex. "You are so beautiful and I love you and desire you so much" are words that almost every woman would like to hear before the sexual act and that would undoubtedly increase her sexual desire and improve her performance. Sex should be a way to express love, respect, and affection.

Remember that a relationship has a life of its own and must be allowed to grow and change. The couple must not feel threatened by this natural phenomenon, but instead, should look at it positively, as representing growth and maturity; they must not consider it a sign of instability, but rather a step forward, toward a closer and more loving relationship.

Success of Treatment

The success of psychotherapy and/or sex therapy for ED is influenced by numerous personal, psychosocial, and medical factors. These include the partner's health, interest in sex, and motivation for and acceptance of treatment; the quality of the overall relationship; the interval of abstinence; and concurrent life stresses, to name a few.

Combined modern psychological and medical treatment is very effective, often yielding excellent results and great couple satisfaction. Using one of the PDE-5 inhibitors may catalyze rapid progress during concurrent psychological treatment and may also improve the man's confidence and bolster his self-esteem. This combination targets the physical and mental disturbances that are often both responsible for ED and produce better results than either mode of therapy alone. Unfortunately, only about 20% of patients with psychogenic ED would accept to consult a psychiatrist. However, the majority of them may still respond to PDE-5 inhibitors or to the intrapenile injections of alprostadil or Trimix injections.

Men who have the best results with sex therapy and psychotherapy for ED are usually those who exhibit strong motivation for this treatment, strong sexual desire, and mutual physical attraction with their partner. They are also those men without any significant psychopathology; those with a sexual disorder of less than two years' duration; and especially those who exhibit early, firm compliance with therapeutic instructions and assignments (Turnbull JM, Weinberg PC 1983). Moreover, the absence of sexual disturbance in the partner and the quality of the couple's relationship—especially the partner's relationship satisfaction—are important factors in success.

Success rates are lowest in young men with marked psychological disturbances, men who lack motivation and confidence in any therapy, and especially men who refuse to admit that their ED is purely psychogenic.

At up to five years of follow-up after the use of sensate focus and sex therapy, Masters and Johnson (1970) reported failure rates of only 41% and 21% for lifelong and acquired sexual dysfunctions, respectively. Their results, however, were not entirely corroborated. Several researchers reported lower success rates of 20% to 30% using the same techniques. Although one study combining modified sex therapy and behavioral systems couples therapy reported improved sexual function in 87% of cases (Wylie KR 1997), others reported long-term success rates varying from 20% to 80%, depending on the factors described previously.

Unfortunately, several problems stand in the way of obtaining accurate, objective reports on the results of these treatment methods. Major deficiencies in the existing studies include small sample size, lack of control groups or standardized definitions, short follow-up, overlapping diagnoses, and narrow or obscure definitions of success (Althof 2005). More randomized, prospective, controlled investigations (as described in chapter 10) are needed to reach proper conclusions regarding the efficacy of sex therapy and psychotherapy for psychogenic ED.

IS PSYCHOLOGICAL REFERRAL ALWAYS NECESSARY?

For some men whose psychogenic ED is clearly due to performance anxiety or mild depression, there is no need for referral to a psychologist or psychiatrist. Such cases of ED involving only minor psychological disturbance may be assessed and treated by a urologist. A few sessions of sex therapy, in addition to pharmacotherapy with a PDE-5 inhibitor, as mentioned, may yield good results. In some cases of minor psychological disturbances with a trial of PDE-5 inhibitors or intracorporeal injections without sex therapy, the success rate may reach about 80%.

However, for patients who have major psychological disorders or for those for whom pharmacotherapy has failed—especially young men—a referral to an expert psychologist or psychiatrist is warranted. In these cases, the best results are usually obtained with traditional psychotherapy, "plus cognitive and interpersonal systems therapy, behavioral assignments, sensate focus, sex education, systematic desensitization, communication and skills training, masturbation exercises, and relapse prevention" (Althof SE et al. 2003, 199).

Chapter Fifteen

EJACULATORY DISORDERS

Sex is the short-cut to everything.

Anne Cunning

Male sexual problems are not limited to erectile dysfunction (ED). Among the other dysfunctions particular to men is the family of ejaculatory disorders, including premature, delayed, and absent ejaculation. In fact, premature ejaculation (PE) is the most common sexual disorder in men aged 18–60. With a worldwide prevalence of about 30%, PE constitutes about 21% of all male sexual disturbances, compared to about 5% for ED.

Only about 10% of men with PE seek medical help, however, so its true prevalence may be much higher than 30%, especially because many men are uncomfortable discussing sex—even with their doctors—out of embarrassment, indifference, or ignorance. And in several cultures (e.g., some parts of Africa, the Middle East, and the Far East), only the man's sexual pleasure matters, so those men who ejaculate quickly most likely do not care and are not inclined to acknowledge it.

PHYSIOLOGY OF EJACULATION

The physiology of normal ejaculation is a complex reflex response to neurobiological and neurobiochemical stimulation. As detailed in chapter 4, neurological regulation of the male human sexual response occurs in the brain and in the thoracolumbar and sacral segments of the spinal cord. The neurotransmitters dopamine and serotonin play a major role in controlling the ejaculatory reflex. Serotonin, acting on 5-HT receptors, is the principal neurotransmitter that inhibits ejaculation; the brain's level of serotonin usually corresponds to a man's ejaculatory latency. Neurons controlled by other chemicals, such as adrenaline, acetylcholine, oxytocin, and aminobutyric acid, may also contribute to the ejaculatory process.

Following the male's maximum arousal and full erection, and with continuing sexual stimulation, the following rapid sequence of events culminates in ejaculation:

Sexual sensations perceived in the hypothalamus and pleasurable stimulation of the penis result in signals being sent via the pudendal and dorsal nerves and sacral spinal cord to the sympathetic intermediolateral columns in the thoracic and lumbar spine at the level of T10–L2.

Return (efferent) signals are transmitted from the spinal cord via the hypogastric and pelvic nerves to the pelvic plexus.

This stimulates neurons called alpha-adrenergic receptors to contract the epididymi, vasa deferentia, seminal vesicles, and prostate, causing emission of these organs' secretions into the posterior urethra after closure of the vesical neck (bladder outlet) and the urethral external sphincter. The sudden distension of the posterior urethra makes ejaculation inevitable.

Onuf's nucleus, the sex center in the sacral spine (nerves S2–S4, specifically), emits additional sympathetic signals. As a result, the urethral external sphincter relaxes, the pudendal nerves cause the pelvic floor and the bulbo- and ischiocavernous muscles surrounding the urethra to contract rhythmically, and ejaculation occurs, forcibly expelling semen out through the urethra.

Orgasm, a pleasurable sensory experience perceived in the brain, usually accompanies ejaculation in the male; orgasm can occur, however, without erection, emission, or ejaculation. Orgasm may also be absent.

Following ejaculation, the male loses his erection and goes through a refractory period, during which no penile tumescence can occur. Depending on his age and other biological and psychosocial factors, and with renewed sexual stimulation, he will then be able to achieve a new erection within a few minutes, hours, or days.

PREMATURE EJACULATION

The consideration of ejaculation's timing is centuries old. The ancient Hindu sex manual *Kama Sutra* and the 1637 Chinese text *Yizong Bidu* (Primer of Medical Objectives), for example, both stress the importance of delaying ejaculation in preventing sexual frustration and reaching a "sexual balance" between man and woman. In 1887, a physician reported the first case of PE in the Western medical literature. Subsequent etiological proposals for the condition involved neurosis, psychosomatic disorder, and neurobiological dysfunction.

Early twentieth-century psychoanalytic theory about PE focused on men's unconscious conflicts about women. Somatic theory, on the other hand, stressed anatomical characteristics such as hyperesthesia (increased sensitivity of the glans penis); a short frenulum (foreskin); or pathologic lesions in the urethra or near the verumontanum (a prominent crest in the urethra, containing the openings of the ejaculatory ducts). As a result, PE was often treated with local anesthetic ointment and electrocautry, which involves cauterizing tissue with an electric current. Note, however, that no reported study has found a difference in the incidence of PE between circumcised and uncircumcised men.

From 1950 to the early 1990s, Masters and Johnson's learned behavior theory was the most accepted explanation for PE's development. It stipulates that the practice of rapid sexual intercourse—in backseats of cars, for example, or due to fear of pregnancy—leads to acquiring the habit of quick ejaculation and becomes coupled with performance anxiety.

The 1990s brought dramatic changes in our understanding of the neurovascular mechanisms underlying the human sexual response. Scientists further elucidated the effects of brain neurotransmitters and the lumbosacral sympathetic nervous system in the erectile and ejaculatory processes. The fortuitous observation of delayed ejaculation as a side effect of some antidepressants contributed to a better understanding of ejaculation's neurological underpinnings and improved pharmacotherapy for PE (University of South Carolina 2005).

Despite these recent advances, PE's pathophysiology is still unknown. It may be a combination of an abnormal serotonin-mediated ejaculatory center in the brain with physical triggers such as inflammation of the urethra or prostate, drug abuse, or excessive efforts to develop an erection—as in an ED patient, for example. A theory proposed by Dr. Waldinger and colleagues (2005) attributes PE to hyposensitivity of 5HT2c receptors or hypersensitivity of 5HT1a receptors in the brain, along with a low concentration of serotonin in the central nervous system. They posit that this combination may either lower a man's ejaculatory threshold, leading to PE, or raise it, resulting in delayed ejaculation.

Other potential risk factors for developing PE include poor general health, lack of sexual experience, infrequent intercourse, and ignorance of the physiological sexual response. At a recent meeting of the American Urological Society, Dr. Stanley Althof also emphasized that the usual psychological response to PE—distress, lack of confidence, depression, embarrassment, anxiety, avoidance of sexual relationships, and preoccupation with sexual functioning—perpetuates and worsens the condition.

Definitions

Several definitions for PE have been proposed, including ejaculation before or within 30 seconds, one minute, or two minutes after penetration, but these criteria have not been universally accepted. The medical community has generally adopted the American Psychiatric Association's (1994) description in the fourth edition of the *Diagnostic and Statistical Manual of Mental Disorders (DSM-IV):*

> Persistent or recurrent ejaculation with minimal sexual stimulation before, upon, or shortly after penetration and before the person wishes it.... The disturbance must cause marked distress or interpersonal difficulty.... The PE is not due exclusively to the direct effects of a substance (e.g., withdrawal from opioids).

This *DSM-IV* definition encompasses not only the time from penetration to ejaculation (normal values of which are still controversial), but also the devastating psychological impact of this condition on the affected man's quality of life and relationship with his partner. The American Urological Association's definition, proposed in 2004, is similar: "Premature ejaculation is ejaculation that occurs sooner than desired, either before or shortly after penetration, causing distress to either one or both partners" (Montague DK et al. 2004). The common threads in most definitions of PE are lack of ejaculatory control, ejaculation much quicker than desired, and its psychological effect on the man or couple, resulting in poor sexual satisfaction. Recently, several experts have considered any ejaculation occurring less than one minute following the development of full erection as premature. However, this definition is not yet widely accepted.

Unfortunately, subjective terminology like "shortly after" or "sooner than desired" creates confusion in PE's identification and management. This vagueness is compounded by lack of consensus on the time to use as a diagnostic criterion, which ranges in published reports from less than one minute to seven minutes. Intravaginal ejaculatory time (IVELT; the total time of vaginal penetration prior to ejaculation) is normally between five and seven minutes, with a mean of nine minutes in healthy men. In a study involving 1,346 men who reported "quick ejaculation," about 63% ejaculated in less than 30 seconds, 77% in less than 60 seconds, and about 6% even before penetration (Waldinger MD et al. 1998; Waldinger MD, Schweitzer DH 2006). The perceived normal time to ejaculation also differs among men from different countries: 13.6 minutes in the United States, 9.9 in the United Kingdom, 9.3 in France, 6.9 in Germany—and these perceptions do not always correspond to somewhat accepted medical norms (Porst H et al. 2006).

Clearly couples' perceptions of PE vary widely; that is, what may be perceived as quick ejaculation by one couple may be considered normal by another. This has led some researchers to define PE not in actual minutes but as a "condition of perception involving poor confidence, low sexual satisfaction, or unrealistic expectations" (Dean J et al. 2005). Because men who ejaculate rapidly are not a homogeneous group, an optimal definition of PE would include an objective measurement of ejaculatory latency, the loss of voluntary control over ejaculation, the presence of interpersonal disturbance, the marked distress produced for the man or couple, and the exclusion of causal factors such as opiate withdrawal (Barada J, McCullough AR 2004, McMahon CG et al. 2004, Sotomayer M et al. 2005).

Causes and Contributors

According to the National Health and Social Life Survey, men with poor to fair health or suffering from stress or emotional problems have a higher incidence of PE. Like ED, PE can be defined as primary, meaning that the man has had it all his life (though he may not have known until he began having sexual intercourse), or secondary, meaning that it followed a period of normal functioning. Primary PE is usually attributed to abnormalities in the brain's 5HT receptors, whereas secondary PE is usually attributed to psychological factors and is usually associated with ED (Sharlip ID 2006). Recent studies suggest, however, that both primary and secondary PE are multifactorial, with overlapping physical, psychological, and contextual etiologies.

The Major Speculative Biological Causes of PE

Disturbed secretion of brain neurotransmitters (namely, serotonin)
Hypersensitivity of the glans, hyperexcitability of the ejaculatory reflex, or sexual Hyperarousability
Poor health
Genetic predisposition (PE is prevalent in certain families and more common among first-degree relatives)
ED, prostatitis, urethritis, or endocrinopathies such as diabetes
Thyroid hyperactivity

The Major Psychological Factors in PE

Sexual inexperience
Stress or anxiety disorders
Infrequent intercourse or complete abstinence
Guilt, fear of failure, or interpersonal conflicts
Early sexual experiences

Additional causal factors in PE are fear of pregnancy or venereal disease, ineffective ejaculatory control techniques, spinal cord injury, alcoholism, inadequate understanding of the sexual response, surgery, and certain prescribed medications, most commonly, some antipsychotics, antidepressants, narcotics, antihypertensives, sedatives, and 5-alpha reductase inhibitors (for benign prostate enlargement). As noted, PE is also a frequent symptom of withdrawal from recreational drugs (McMahon CG et al. 2004).

It is important to consider that some patients with ED may end up with PE as well because their aggressive and overzealous efforts to achieve an erection can lead to rapid orgasm and ejaculation. Conversely, many men with PE can subsequently develop ED because of high performance anxiety, fear of failure, their partner's negative reaction, depression, and/or other psychogenic disturbances (see the following discussion).

Emotional Effects on the Man and the Couple

Some people might argue that the concept of prematurity in ejaculation could simply represent a natural process, rather than a problem. Several animals, among them the king of the jungle, engage in several successive intercourses, each time ejaculating within a few seconds after intromission. This pattern serves the goal of preservation, as the lion risks attack by other predators if he indulges in lengthy sexual intercourse, during which he may be unable to defend himself. Even elephants ejaculate quickly usually within one minute. For humans, however, rapid ejaculation may be emotionally devastating, especially if the man cares about his partner's sexual satisfaction, or if the partner suffers and complains about deprivation of sexual pleasure (Patrick DC et al. 2005). A woman's sexual response cycle is usually much slower than her male partner's, and it may take her 10–20 minutes to reach orgasm, compared to 2–10 minutes for a man.

Unfortunately, in various parts of the world, women still accept their traditional role as providers of pleasure for men, without considering their own sexual satisfaction and without the courage, or sometimes even the right, to complain or object. As I was once told by a Middle Eastern woman who had never experienced orgasm, "I feel like an ATM machine. My husband inserts his card [penis] in the slot, gets his money [orgasm], and good-bye and thank you…and all this within two to three minutes.…The faster the better!" For this kind of man, PE is not a problem, as long as he can have his own pleasure. And for a large number of women who are not interested in sex, PE is of no consequence either.

But for the majority of men and women who want to share their sexual pleasure and strive for mutual sexual satisfaction, PE may lead to devastating emotional disturbances (Patrick DL et al. 2006). The patient with PE often suffers from anxiety about sex, low self-esteem, and feelings of inferiority, depression, a sense of failure, embarrassment, and shame for not being able to satisfy his partner. These negative emotions may affect his highly prized sense of virility and manhood and strain the relationship.

Other emotional reactions involve frustration, anger, suspicion, jealousy, and guilt—and the partner's misperception of the affected man's sexual selfishness. Ensuing dire consequences for both people can be dissatisfaction with intercourse, generation of numerous excuses to avoid sexual communication or contact, and difficulty initiating or maintaining relationships. The man may ultimately avoid sex altogether or end up with ED, while the woman may subsequently develop sexual difficulties herself. In most cases, the price of PE is the abrupt end of intimacy.

NEWSFLASH: PARTNERS' PERCEPTIONS OF PREMATURE EJACULATION

Perceptions of premature ejaculation's (PE) presence or absence may differ between the man and his sexual partner. In a recent study (Patrick DL et al. 2006), self-reported measures of ejaculatory control, general distress, sexual satisfaction, and interpersonal difficulty were, not surprisingly, worse in the PE couples than the non-PE couples; but interestingly, the women in both groups reported better perceptions of the men's control and lower levels of distress than the men did. In another survey of female partners of men with PE (Rosenberg MT et al. 2006), only 23% of the women reported lessened sexual satisfaction; about 65%, however, reported an interest in treatment.

Diagnosis

An accurate diagnosis based on careful analysis of the various potential biological or psychosocial factors in ejaculatory dysfunction can generally be achieved by taking a meticulous medical and sexual history, followed by a proper physical examination, as detailed in chapter 7. When PE is suspected, the most important facets of the sexual history are estimated intravaginal latency prior to ejaculation, duration and origin of the problem, any difficulty achieving or maintaining erection, degree of desire, frequency of rapid ejaculation, and its effect on the man and the couple. Questions about quality and duration of erections, ejaculatory control, frequency of intercourse, history of prostatitis or thyroid disease, and pain in either partner during or after sex are also helpful. Additional questions should address both partners' degree of sexual satisfaction and level of distress as well as their desire to correct the problem. It behooves the physician to make all of these inquiries tactfully, but also very thoroughly.

For the sake of effective treatment, it is extremely important to differentiate between PE and ED, as the two conditions may occur together, or the patient himself may mix them up. Some men with PE, for example, erroneously consider their loss of erection after rapid ejaculation to represent ED. The physician must question the patient carefully to determine whether ejaculation or the sensation of ejaculation occurs before the loss of erection, which would support the diagnosis of PE.

Unfortunately, about 90% of men who experience ejaculatory disturbance refuse to volunteer any information about it, unless a physician specifically quizzes them; even then, most are not receptive to any investigation or therapy for it. The causes of this voluntary omission include the associated stigma, embarrassment, shyness, and reluctance to discuss intimate problems. False beliefs about PE range from the notion that it is only temporary and corrects itself spontaneously to the idea that all cases are psychological and that no treatment is successful. Some affected men disregard their partners' sexual needs; others argue that, because their partners do not complain, or can reach orgasm themselves within a few minutes, there is nothing of concern.

The physical exam should focus on signs of chronic illness and endocrine dysfunction, secondary sexual characteristics, neurologic assessment, and palpation of the testicles and penis for abnormalities. Checking the chest for gynecomastia (breast enlargement), the urethra for urethritis, and the prostate for infection are also important for discovering possible etiologic factors.

Treatment Options

It is quite unfortunate that only about 12% of men with PE seek medical help or accept treatment. The majority tend to either ignore the condition or use self-taught, generally unsuccessful methods to deal with it. One of the most common techniques is masturbation before sex, which may delay subsequent ejaculation in some cases but which risks, especially in elderly men, a long refractory period before achieving a second erection. Other methods include mental distraction during sex, wearing several condoms to decrease glans sensitivity, forceful and rapid thrusting to quicken the partner's orgasm, spraying the glans with anesthetic, or using over-the-counter herbal desensitization ointments. Most of these techniques are doomed to failure because controlling ejaculation requires awareness of sexual sensations. Control can, however, be achieved by certain behavioral, pharmacological, or mechanical means.

The primary goal of PE treatment is to help the couple achieve physical, subjective, and emotional satisfaction in sex. Any therapy should focus not only on the man, but also on his partner and their lovemaking process. It is not enough to teach a man exercises or to prescribe medication without considering the effects of the couple's relationship and sexual behavior on his PE. Careful inquiry regarding the partner's low desire or lack of interest in sex may sometimes even reveal satisfaction with the patient's quick ejaculation and a total disinterest in any type of therapy.

Administration of any therapy for PE must provide not only efficacy, but also safety. The patient must understand all potential hazards and benefits prior to acceptance. Current options include behavioral therapy, psychotherapy, and pharmacotherapy. Most men suffering from PE select pharmacotherapy as their first option. I must emphasize that any pharmacotherapy—oral or topical—must be initiated and followed under strict, expert medical supervision to prevent serious side effects.

Behavioral Therapy and Psychotherapy

At the American Urological Association's 2006 annual meeting, in a debate on the optimal treatment for PE, psychologist Stanley Althof argued for behavioral psychotherapy. Although he conceded that pharmacotherapy is often successful, he pointed out that it does not address the multiple psychosocial issues related to PE, which also have to be managed for the patient to regain his self-esteem and sexual confidence and to relieve his performance anxiety. In addition to enhancing the couple's satisfaction in their sexual relationship, psychotherapy also offers a safe and successful way to deal with the multiple psychological disturbances associated with PE. Dr. Althof reported that short-term success rates from a recent series of treatment studies with behavioral therapy ranged from 64% to 80%. However, very few reports of this treatment's long-term results appear in the literature, and those that do have a success rate of only about 25% (De Amicis LA et al. 1985). In some selected patients, the best results are obtained by the combination of psychotherapy and pharmacology.

In 1956, psychologist Dr. Semans introduced the stop-and-start method. It consists of manual, sexual penile stimulation that is suddenly discontinued when the man feels the imminent approach of ejaculation. When this premonitory sensation passes, the stimulation is resumed, and the same procedure of stop and start is repeated. After three or four successive trials, he is allowed to reach orgasm. The patient and couple practice the stop-and-start method with manual penile stimulation for several weeks. As they become more confident in the man's control of his ejaculation, they proceed to intercourse, applying the stop-and-start method during sex (Semans JH 1959). This method is helpful in the management of some cases of PE.

In 1970, Masters and Johnson presented the squeeze technique, in which the patient and his partner are taught to squeeze forcibly at the base of the glans for about three to four seconds when the patient feels the urge to ejaculate. This not only delays ejaculation, but also teaches awareness of the sensations that precede it so that its timing can be controlled. The technique is first applied by the patient for about two weeks during self-masturbation. When he becomes more confident in controlling his ejaculation, sexual intercourse is resumed, with his partner squeezing the glans when the man feels the approaching orgasm. The couple then progresses from intercourse with the woman positioned on top, with no or minimal thrusting or movement of the penis in the vagina, to assuming the lateral face-to-face position, with both partners moving; in both positions, they are to interrupt the sex act with the squeeze technique when ejaculation feels imminent. Masters and Johnson (1970) initially reported an immediate 99% success rate with this technique; however, subsequent studies with longer follow-up yielded much lower success rates.

Other behavioral strategies for PE treatment include sensate focus (described in chapter 14), anxiety-relieving techniques, psychotherapy, hypnosis, relaxation exercises, and marriage/relationship counseling. Deep muscle relaxation, education, and reassurance are additional helpful tools in the couple's sexual rehabilitation. Most of these behavioral therapies, which may be necessary and efficacious, especially in cases of secondary PE, which occur following a period of normal ejaculation, require great dedication and close cooperation on the part of the couple for successful results, so most men with PE prefer newer, simpler, and sometimes more effective pharmacological treatments.

Oral Medications

Surprisingly, some antidepressant drugs have found an additional application in the treatment of PE. Unexpected clinical observations that patients taking certain antidepressants complained of delayed or absent ejaculation were consonant with the finding that PE may be associated with a decrease in the brain's concentration of serotonin. As a result, tricyclic antidepressants and selective serotonin reuptake inhibitors (SSRIs), which increases cerebral serotonin by inhibiting its reuptake, have been used extensively in PE's management. The first trials of paroxetine for PE began in 1994. Paroxetine and its fellow SSRIs fluoxetine, sertraline, citalopram, and fluvoxamine are the antidepressants now most commonly used for PE, with paroxetine the most successful (Rivera P et al. 2005). Another antidepressant, clomipramine, is also successful but is associated with a high incidence of adverse reactions (5% to 15%).

These drugs are taken on demand three to six hours before sexual intercourse, or continuously in a reduced dose for three to six weeks, and then in a full dose a few hours before sex. With the on-demand method, intravaginal latency to ejaculation (timed with a stopwatch) is three to nine minutes, compared to less than one minute for the patients taking placebo tablets. With the daily dose for four to six weeks followed by the presex dose, latency increases as much as 10-fold, from 3 to 10 minutes with the medication compared to less than 1 to 2 minutes with placebo.

The SSRIs require a prolonged time (4.5–8 hours) to achieve maximum concentration in the bloodstream, which may be responsible for their slowness of action, and a positive response may take two to three weeks to manifest itself (Sharlip ID 2006). Therefore a daily dosing schedule may be more effective for PE, even though on-demand use is better accepted by patients. But another limitation is that side effects are associated with SSRIs' long half-lives (20–36 hours). Significant adverse reactions—especially at higher doses—include nausea, vomiting, dry mouth, drowsiness, reduced potency, diminished desire, absent ejaculation, reduction in penile rigidity, mania, and sensory confusion as well as withdrawal symptoms if the medication is stopped abruptly. There is a rare risk of suicide associated with these medications.

Nevertheless, these drugs have been recommended by the American Urological Association's panel of experts and incorporated in that organization's treatment guidelines for PE (Montague DK et al. 2004). The panel stated that the optimal treatment should be based on the physician's discretion and the patient's preference and that when ED and PE occur together, as happens in about 30% of men with sexual dysfunction, ED should be treated first.

The phosphodiesterase type 5 (PDE-5) inhibitors, used alone or in combination with one of the aforementioned SSRIs, have also shown some effectiveness against PE, especially when associated with ED. In a study of combined treatment with Viagra and paroxetine, intravaginal latency time for the treated group was about 4.5 minutes versus about 35 seconds for the placebo group. The treated group also experienced greater sexual satisfaction, albeit an increased incidence of adverse reactions such as headaches and flushing (Salonia A et al. 2002). In another study, Levitra alone prolonged preejaculatory latency for as long as or longer than Zoloft did (Susman ED 2005). These results have been attributed to the relief of anxiety over losing the erection and needing to rush to orgasm, or to a central effect such as allowing the development of erection with less sexual stimulation (Sharlip ID 2006). However, a recent review of 14 studies failed to demonstrate any benefit of PDE-5 inhibitors alone or combined with SSRIs for acquired PE combined with ED (McMahon CG et al. 2006).

Ideally, oral pharmacotherapy for PE should be simple, safe, on-demand, fast acting, specific to the PE-related serotonin receptors, and highly effective within a short period. A new serotonin modulator called dapoxetine, specifically developed for PE, fits this description. Preliminary studies showed dapoxetine was rapidly absorbed, reaching maximum concentration in only 1.5–2 hours. It prolonged intravaginal latency from 0.98 minutes to 3.10 minutes (216%), with great patient satisfaction and significantly improved couples' satisfaction. Nausea occurred in about 8.5% to 20% of cases, depending on dose, with headache in about 6% and diarrhea in about 6%. The dropout rate due to side effects was 4% for the 30-milligram dose and 10% for the 60-milligram dose. U.S. Food and Drug Administration (FDA) approval of dapoxetine would open new horizons in PE treatment.

Another potential drug which may have great potential in the treatment of PE is Tramadol HCL, which is an opiate agonist used for the management of moderate to severe pain. When used in a dose of 25 milligrams one to two hours before sexual intercourse, it prolonged the IVELT from about 1.17 minutes before treatment to about 7.35 minutes after its use (Salem EA et al. 2007). It certainly needs further study to assess its efficacy.

Topical Anesthetics and Other Medications

Among the various topical creams and gels used to desensitize the glans, the most popular is EMLA cream, which contains two local anesthetics, lidocaine 2.5 % and prilocaine 2.5 %. A spray (TEMPE) containing these two anesthetics—lidocaine 7.5 mg and prilocaine 2.5 mg—has been recently introduced in the United States. It is applied on the glans 20–30 minutes prior to intercourse, with the optional use of a condom to keep the cream applied for this period, and then thoroughly washed off before sex to prevent numbness of the glans or desensitization of the partner's vagina. Several studies have confirmed the effectiveness of the EMLA cream, or of the same anesthetic combination in a spray, in prolonging ejaculatory latency. Its major drawback is numbness if applied for an extended period. In a similar vein, a recent study from Turkey demonstrated superior response to a combination of fluoxetine (taken orally four hours before sex) and lidocaine ointment (applied 20 minutes before sex) over fluoxetine alone in prolonging ejaculatory latency, with minimal side effects (Metin A et al. 2005).

SS cream, manufactured in Korea and not yet FDA approved, contains nine different herbs. Its mode of action is still obscure, although a few Korean studies attribute it to desensitization of the glans and decreased hyperexcitability; it may also have a local anesthetic effect. When SS cream was applied for about one hour before intercourse and then washed off, prolongation of IVELT was about 10–13 minutes, compared to 2.4 minutes for the placebo. Mild burning and pain in the glans were reported in about 18% of cases but disappeared within one hour, and no other local or systemic adverse reactions were noted. Prospective, well-controlled, randomized, international studies are warranted to assess the efficacy and safety of SS cream.

Additional Types of Treatment

If behavioral therapy, psycholotherapy, and pharmacotherapy are unsuccessful or refused by the patient or couple, or in cases of significant adverse reactions, two other therapeutic options for PE can be adapted from ED treatments. Use of a vacuum pump allows the man to maintain his erection even after ejaculation, as long as the constrictive ring remains at the base of the penis. Decreased sympathetic nervous system activity prolongs preejaculatory latency, reducing ejaculatory anxiety and giving the partner an opportunity to achieve sexual satisfaction. Another method of maintaining erection even after quick ejaculation or orgasm is the intracorporeal injection of vasodilators. (Pumps and injections are detailed in chapter 12.)

Other maneuvers that may be successful in managing PE include pelvic muscle exercises, with rapid and slow contractions of the external urethral sphincter three times daily to strengthen it. When the man feels the approach of orgasm during intercourse, he can rapidly contract the sphincter, inhibiting orgasm and ejaculation. This allows him to control his ejaculation at will and enjoy prolonged sexual activity. A more sophisticated variant of this method, which could provide excellent results, consists of home exercises involving masturbation with sensate focus provided by caressing the erogenic spots in the body, including the penis. With the approach of ejaculation, all caresses are stopped, and the man expires deeply and then takes deep breaths while contracting his external urethral sphincter (the pubococcygeal muscles) and, holding his breath, then contracts other muscles, including those of the thighs, the back, the shoulders, the biceps, the hands, the abdomen, and the jaw. He maintains his muscular contractions for 10 seconds, and then he relaxes them, while expiring and breathing deeply and normally. He will experience orgasm without ejaculation and will lose his erection, to regain it again with foreplay (Brissard E 2006).

ABSENT EJACULATION

As mentioned in chapter 3, a man's ejaculated fluid, which usually measures 1.5–4.5 milliliters, originates mainly from the seminal vesicles, which contribute 50% to 70% of the total ejaculate volume. The rest comes from the prostate (15% to 30% of ejaculate volume) and the ampulla of the vasa deferentia (less than 5%). Absence of ejaculation during sexual intercourse may be physically and psychologically distressing, especially if it affects the ability to conceive. When no seminal fluid is ejected from the body despite the occurrence of orgasm, three underlying mechanisms are most likely: retrograde (backward) ejaculation of semen into the bladder, defective production of semen, or obstruction of the ejaculatory ducts.

Retrograde passage of semen usually results from failure of the bladder's neck to close during ejaculation. This may be caused by peripheral neuropathy due to diabetes, previous resection or incision of the bladder neck, excision of an aortic aneurysm, or para-aortic lymphadenectomy. Other causes of retrograde ejaculation include some neurogenic conditions, medications such as alpha-blockers, or transection of the sympathetic nerves during surgery or trauma.

Anejaculation, or the complete lack of ejaculation in either direction, may be due to inadequate production of seminal fluid by the seminal vesicles and prostate, congenital anomalies of the vasa deferentia and seminal vesicles, or pituitary and testicular deficiencies leading to low concentrations of luteinizing hormone and testosterone. Obstruction of the ejaculatory ducts—for example, by congenital cysts, a chronic genitourinary infection such as tuberculosis or schistosomiasis, scarring from radiation therapy, or prostatic calculi (stones)—is another major cause. Obstruction is commonly diagnosed by transrectal ultrasonography of the prostate and the ejaculatory ducts.

Other Physical Factors in Anejaculation

Defective sympathetic nervous stimulation that inhibits contractions of the vasa
   deferentia and seminal vesicles
Surgical excision of the prostate and seminal vesicles for prostate cancer
Spinal cord injury
A case of prune belly syndrome (characterized by lax, wrinkled suprapubic skin;
   dilated bladder, ureters, and parts of the kidneys; and undescended testicles)
Rarely, diminished secretion of thyroid hormone
Surgical excision of the colon and rectum
Certain medications such as alpha methyldopa, thiazide diuretics, various antide-
   pressants, and phenothiazine

Alcohol and Drug Abuse

Psychological, behavioral, and interrelationship factors inhibiting ejaculation may include religious orthodoxy, fear of pregnancy, overdominance of the mother, homosexuality, past traumatic events, and vaginal aversion. Misconceptions and poor sex education, resentment toward the partner, desire for punitive revenge, or subconscious transposition of the mother's image on the female partner (with apprehension of soiling her vagina) may play a major role in some cases of anejaculation or retarded ejaculation.

To differentiate between retrograde and completely absent ejaculation, a careful physical exam with palpation of the vasa, seminal vesicles, and prostate is very helpful. A urine test may be conducted, following masturbation or intercourse, for the presence of fructose (secreted by the seminal vesicles) and sperms; if present, these confirm the diagnosis of retrograde ejaculation.

Treatment and Fertility Issues

The primary treatment for retrograde ejaculation is the use of oral medications such as midodrin, imipramine, pseudoephedrine, or chlorpropamine and other sympathomimetics, which help close the bladder's neck during ejaculation. If these drugs fail and the patient is interested in conception, his seminal fluid can be retrieved with a catheter from the bladder (following intercourse or masturbation) for placement into his partner's cervix, uterus, or fallopian tubes. In rare cases, the bladder's neck can be surgically closed.

Anejaculation due to defective activity of the sympathetic nervous system can be treated with sympathomimetic drugs but this usually yields poor results. For conception purposes, application of a penile vibrator to the glans or frenulum, or introduction of an electrical instrument in the rectum to stimulate the nerves around the prostate and seminal vesicles, can produce ejaculation to obtain viable sperms for insemination. If these techniques are unsuccessful, sperms can be aspirated by needle from the epididymis or testicle and injected into eggs retrieved from the woman's ovary for intracytoplasmic sperm insemination and fertilization, followed by transfer of the embryo to the uterus after approximately three days.

In cases of obstruction of the ejaculatory ducts by a large intraprostatic cyst, surgical resection of the cyst or aspiration of sperms from the seminal vesicles for insemination in the partner's cervix or uterus may help achieve pregnancy. If absent ejaculation is secondary to obstruction of the ejaculatory ducts by fibrosis, such as following radiotherapy to the prostate, the use of one of the PDE-5 inhibitors (Viagra, Cialis, or Levitra) in combination with a smooth muscle relaxant, such as yohimbine or alfuzocin, may help, in some cases, to restore ejaculation.

DELAYED EJACULATION

A delay in ejaculation, with occasional absent or diminished orgasm (see the following discussion), is usually caused by an inhibition of the ejaculatory reflex, due mainly to psychological factors. Delayed ejaculation is called "global" if it occurs in all instances of sexual intercourse or "situational" if it happens only under specific circumstances or with particular partners.

Beside the psychological inhibitors listed previously, high-frequency masturbation (especially using idiosyncratic means), old age, lack of physical attraction to the partner, repressed homosexual tendencies, past traumatic events, inhibited arousal, successive sexual intercourses, and relationship disturbances are additional etiological factors. Other contributors include misconceptions and ignorance about the genital organs and proper sexual functioning. Rarely, biological factors such as neurologic disease or the use of medications such as PDE-5 inhibitors, antiandrogens, antiadrenergic agents, antidepressants, antipsychotics, and sedatives may cause ejaculatory delay.

The management of delayed ejaculation is often difficult and not very successful, except when the medications responsible can be discontinued or when reversible behavioral or psychological causes are identified and treated by an expert. Counseling directed at limiting the frequency of masturbation and refraining from idiosyncratic masturbatory methods may help a large number of patients. In addition, sex therapy and psychotherapy may assist in curtailing the psychological inhibitions that delay ejaculation. This includes sex education to dispel misconceptions, relieve anxieties and fears, and eliminate apprehension about hurting the partner. Therapy may also involve helping the individual to detach from his mother so he can commit himself to another woman.

Additional measures include teaching the patient how to focus on the pleasurable sensations associated with manual stimulation of the penis and instructing him to indulge in sexual fantasies and superstimulation techniques (such as with a vibrator or high-speed water jet from a showerhead on the glans and frenulum, or the use of oils) during masturbation and foreplay. He is encouraged to use self-masturbation in the presence of his partner, who may later assist in stimulating his penis. It is only when the man feels confident and capable of ejaculation that penetration and ejaculation during intercourse are resumed.

Several medications, namely, the sympathomimetics (drugs that stimulate the sympathetic nervous system), have been used to treat delayed ejaculation, but with limited success. In selected cases of ejaculatory delay or absent orgasm (see the following discussion) with poor sexual desire and with or without ED secondary to an SSRI antidepressant, replacement of the SSRI with Wellbutrin (bupropion), buspirone, amantadine, or cyproheptadine may yield good results.

ANORGASMIA

Ejaculation can occur in the absence of orgasm. Anorgasmia, or the absence of orgasm, is usually divided into three categories. The primary type involves men who have never experienced an orgasm, the secondary type involves men who fail to achieve orgasm after having had normal orgasms in the past, and the tertiary involves men who complain of undue delay in reaching orgasm during sex or of low-intensity orgasm. A possible fourth category includes men who can have normal orgasm and ejaculation during masturbation but not during sexual intercourse.

Most cases of primary anorgasmia may be caused by neurobiological factors involving dopamine and serotonin pathways in the brain. These factors are attributed to such psychological causes as an overly strict upbringing, religious orthodoxy, homosexuality, poor sexual stimulation, inadequate arousal and poor vaginal lubrication in the female partner, fear of pregnancy or sexually transmitted disease, performance anxiety, and pains in the vagina during intromission. Other familial, social, and cultural influences can also repress the normal response to sexual stimulation. In the second and third categories of anorgasmia, in addition to psychological factors, a neurologic condition, such as spinal cord injury, multiple sclerosis, parkinsonism, or trauma to the pelvic nerves, may contribute to the problem. Furthermore, some antidepressants may affect the intensity of orgasm.

On the other hand, the occurrence of orgasm and ejaculation with masturbation but not with sexual intercourse is caused in the majority of cases by excessive and high-frequency masturbation using idiosyncratic techniques with particular fantasies that cannot be duplicated or achieved during sexual intercourse. More rarely, it may be caused by deep anxiety during coitus, neuropathy of the pudendal or penile dorsal nerve, or a neurologic disease such as multiple sclerosis. Diagnosis relies on a neurologic examination and special emphasis during the sexual history interview on the patient's masturbatory patterns, frequency, and methods, including his fantasies.

The management of anorgasmia is difficult and does not guarantee good results. It consists of psychotherapy, sex therapy, masturbation or intercourse with stimulating devices like a vibrator, and the use of certain medications such as high doses of yohimbine (see chapter 11). In cases caused by SSRI antidepressants like paroxetine, the clinician may suggest replacing the SSRI with another medication such as Wellbutrin (bupropion), amantadine, or cyproheptadine (Ralph DJ, Wylie KR 2005). On the other hand, for anorgasmia due to excessive masturbation, modifying the masturbatory behavior through sex therapy may help a substantial number of patients achieve orgasm and ejaculation during intercourse (Perelman MA 2006). The addition of certain medications, such as BuSpar (buspirone hydrochloride), to relieve anxiety, and others, including yohimbine, Ritalin, and pseudoephedrine for possible action on the brain or sympathetic nervous system, may be beneficial in a few cases.

Chapter Sixteen

LOW SEXUAL DESIRE IN MEN

Sex at age ninety is like trying to shoot pool with a rope.

George Burns

The intensity of sexual desire in healthy men and women differs from one person to the other. Hypoactive desire, which affects millions of people worldwide, is probably the most underestimated, neglected, undefined, difficult to evaluate and treat, and frustrating sexual disorder. Health care providers are faced with a plethora of clinical studies on various other sexual disturbances but with a dearth of evidence regarding the proper diagnosis and management of low sexual desire, no objective tools to assess or measure it, and plenty of misconceptions and ignorance about it. Diminished desire or low libido in men is commonly, and erroneously, misdiagnosed and treated as erectile disorder (ED)—with very poor results in most cases.

Furthermore, all the commonly used so-called aphrodisiac foods, herbs, potions, and concoctions, such as ginseng, Spanish fly, cantharide, caviar, oysters, chocolate, strawberries, spicy foods, Ginkgo biloba, and moderate amounts of alcohol, have not been proven particularly effective. It was suggested recently that nuts could increase sexual desire; however, this claim needs to be substantiated by further scientific studies. In cases when some of the aforementioned substances are successful for increasing libido in some men, perhaps it is because they may block mental sexual inhibitions or work on a motivational or other psychological level.

"VIAGRAVATION"

With the availability and success of the phosphodiesterase type 5 inhibitors in restoring normal sexual functioning, millions of men with erectile dysfunction (ED) can achieve firm, lasting erections allowing satisfactory intercourse. But those medications cannot heighten libido—so, ironically, a large group of men are capable of producing erections but have little or no real desire to do so. Some of them would rather play golf or watch television; many others, however, are frustrated by their low desire and would very much like to experience the ultimate joy of sex once again. Viagravation is a term that was proposed to describe the deep aggravation experienced by men who are willing and able to use an ED medication to achieve erection but lack the physiological or psychological motivation to engage in sex—with the resulting deep frustration experienced by their sexual partners.

THEORIES OF SEXUAL DESIRE

The complex cerebral phenomenon of sexual desire is poorly understood despite various theories of its mechanism. Masters and Johnson (1970) originally proposed the linear theory, which stipulates that "sexual thoughts and fantasies and an innate urge to experience sexual tensions and release are markers of desire." They emphasized that "the personal experience of lustful desire in both sexual partners should precede any initiation of sexuality" (Meuleman EJH, Van Lankveld JDM 2004).

Real life, however, demonstrates universal differences between partners' experiences of sexual desire, for example, in timing and frequency of sexual activity. In addition, couples engage in sexual activity not only because of an intrinsic urge, but also for nonsexual motives such as pleasing the partner, distracting from boredom or gloom, material rewards, or other conjugal or personal reasons; this is termed "receptive sexual desire," as opposed to "active desire." The oversimplified linear model soon gave way to multifactorial or circular hypotheses of interrelationship among sexual desire, arousal, and performance, influenced by unconscious and conscious motives.

Janssen et al.'s (2000) theory of sexual desire presents a two-stage information-processing model. In the first stage, subliminal sexual stimuli, such as subconscious fantasies and thoughts, prepare the sexual system for arousal by rendering it receptive to the perception of additional erotic stimuli such as touch, sight, sound, and odor. Following this primary motivational engagement, the man can become aware of a desire to proceed with the enjoyment of a sexual experience. Thus Janssen et al. propose that an arousal phase precedes and motivates desire.

The mental sexual arousal then modulates the chemicals in the brain's limbic centers, leading to secretion of the facilitating neurotransmitter oxytocin and blocking the inhibiting neurotransmitter serotonin. This process, by activating the sex center in the sacral spinal cord, stimulates the pelvic and penile nerves to produce penile engorgement and erection, which is gratifying and reinforces or increases the man's desire and arousal (Meuleman EJH, Van Lankveld JDM 2004). But during this second stage, it is also possible for inhibitory stimuli, such as mental preoccupation, anxiety, anger, fear of failure, and nonsexual thoughts, to derail the process.

HYPOACTIVE SEXUAL DESIRE

In the *Diagnostic and Statistical Manual of Mental Disorders*, fourth edition (American Psychiatric Association 1994), hypoactive sexual desire disorder (HSDD) is defined as "the persistent or recurrent absence or deficit of sexual fantasies and desire for sexual activity, accounting for factors that affect sexual function, e.g., age, sex, and life context." It is extremely difficult to assess HSSD's true prevalence, which ranges from zero to 15% in population-based studies—this is certainly an underestimation, especially as most men do not reveal sexual problems unless explicitly questioned by their physicians.

Assessment of a libido problem is based on direct and unambiguous questions, posed by the physician to the patient, regarding sexual motivation and desire. Additional helpful information can be obtained from the patient's partner or by using questionnaires such as the Sexual Desire Inventory or the Golombock-Rust Inventory of Sexual Satisfaction.

Hypoactive desire results from a wide variety of biological and psychological factors, including aging and chronic medical conditions such as coronary artery disease (CAD), heart failure, AIDS, and renal failure. Some bodybuilders and men with eating disorders are also subject to low desire. The psychiatric conditions most commonly associated with low libido include depression, anxiety, anger, and relationship disorders (Morales A 2003, Wyllie MG 2003, Meuleman EJH, Van Lankveld JDM 2004, Wyllie MG 2005).

NEWSFLASH: DESIRE IN DNA

Although it has long been accepted that desire in both genders depends on psychological and hormonal factors, no definitive scientific proof has supported this theory. But a study recently published in *Molecular Psychiatry* (Ebstein RP 2006), by examining the DNA of 148 healthy male and female university students, demonstrated that self-reported low sexual desire was correlated with genetic differences, namely, "the variants in a gene called the D4 receptor" (Ebstein RP 2006). This may mean that low sexual desire can be considered a normal biological, rather than psychological, condition. Of course, this interesting finding requires confirmation by additional multicenter studies before its acceptance by the medical community.

Hormonal Etiologies

Hormonal underpinnings of decreased sexual desire are complex. It has long been medically accepted that low serum levels of the male hormone testosterone may result in absent or hypoactive desire in older men as well as in postmenopausal women. In males, this hormone is produced when the brain's hypothalamus secretes gonadotropin-releasing hormone (GnRH), stimulating the pituitary gland to produce two hormones: follicular stimulating hormone (FSH), which contributes to sperm production, and luteinizing hormone (LH), which stimulates the testicles to secrete testosterone. (Most testosterone is produced by the testicles, and some by the adrenal glands.)

Testosterone plays major roles in spermatogenesis, embryonic sexual differentiation (see the sidebar), pubertal maturation, and pituitary gonadotropin secretion. It also affects the body's secretion of erythropoietin (a hormone from the adult kidneys that stimulates bone marrow to produce red blood cells), muscle growth and strength, insulin secretion and sensitivity, serum lipid profile, and blood pressure. It also regulates the formation of cyclic guanosine monophosphate through nitric oxide synthase, which is essential for the development and maintenance of a hard erection. This could explain the poor response to phosphodiesterase type 5 inhibitors in cases of hypogonadism (Morelli A et al. 2007).

In the newborn male, concentrations of serum FSH, LH, and testosterone are low but then rise for several months after birth and decline again by 9–12 months. From six to eight years of age until the completion of puberty, LH and FSH progressively increase, along with a steep rise in testosterone at age 12–14 secondary to the nighttime hypersecretion of LH during midpuberty. Men produce about 5 milligrams of testosterone per day.

Testosterone secretion can be impaired, however, by congenital or pathological lesions in the testicles, pituitary, or hypothalamus. Interference with the hypothalamus or pituitary by elevated blood levels of testosterone, estradiol, or prolactin may also lead to hypoactive or absent sexual desire.

To summarize, the involved endocrine organs and their hormones are as follows:

Hypothalamus: GnRH, other hormones
Pituitary gland: prolactin, secreted by specialized lactotroph cells; LH; FSH; other gonadotropins; human gonadotropin hormone
Testicles: most testosterone (about 90%), secreted by specialized Leydig cells
Adrenal glands: a little testosterone (about 10%), adrenaline, other hormones

---

TESTOSTERONE AND OTHER HORMONES IN UTERO

Sexual differentiation in the fetus occurs after the sixth week of gestation and under the influence of multiple genes, especially the SRY gene on the sex-determining region of the Y chromosome. At this time, the primitive testicles form Leydig cells, Sertoli cells (these provide support, nutrition, and protection to developing sperms), and Mullerian inhibiting substance (MIS). MIS causes regression of the fetal paramesonephric ducts, which would otherwise—in the female, who doesn't produce MIS—form the fallopian tubes, uterus, and upper two-thirds of the vagina.

The formation of testosterone from cholesterol is responsible for development of the male genital ducts, including the vas deferens, epididymis, and seminal vesicles from the fetal mesonephric ducts. Placental luteinizing hormone (LH) prompts the initial secretion of testosterone from the new Leydig cells. Concomitantly in early gestation, the fetal pituitary gland in both males and females begins to synthesize and store its own LH and follicular stimulating hormone and secretes them in high concentrations, contributing to the secretion of testosterone. Starting in the fourth month of gestation, the male external genitalia (penis and scrotum) develop under the influence of dihydrotestosterone, which is converted from testosterone by the enzyme 5-alpha reductase.

Hyperprolactinemia

Elevated serum prolactin is associated with disturbed reproductive functions in both men and women and may directly inhibit some of the brain's sex centers. In men, hyperprolactinemia can inhibit the secretion of GnRH, which normally leads to testicular testosterone production, as described previously. Subsequent symptoms may include loss of sexual desire, ED, infertility, and poor energy. The accompanying low testosterone level may also lead to osteoporosis, hair loss, and loss of muscle mass.

Various diseases and physiological conditions may elevate serum prolactin, most commonly a pituitary adenoma (benign epithelial tumor). Rarely, hyperprolactinemia is due to an increase in the number of lactotrophs in the pituitary or a tumor in or near the hypothalamus. Other causes include drugs that are dopamine receptor antagonists (which nullify the action of dopamine receptors), such as certain antipsychotics, antihypertensives, and antidepressants; hypothyroidism (insufficient activity and hormone secretion of the thyroid gland); and conditions such as chest wall injury or chronic renal failure. But in a substantial number of patients with elevated prolactin, no cause can be found despite an extensive workup.

Diagnosis of hyperprolactinemia relies on a thorough medical history with special emphasis on sexual symptoms as well as any changes in vision or chronic headaches, which may point to a pituitary or brain lesion. A complete physical exam, including the assessment of field of vision, is followed by laboratory evaluation. Serum concentrations of prolactin, testosterone, and other pituitary hormones are measured at least twice, preferably in the morning.

In cases of elevated prolactin, radiological studies via MRI, CT scan, and, rarely, a positron-emission tomography scan may help identify a pituitary adenoma or some other benign or malignant brain tumor.

Management of hyperprolactinemia due to adenoma relies on dopamine-agonist medications, such as cabergoline or bromocriptine, to lower prolactin and raise testosterone. This treatment is usually very successful in restoring sexual desire and improving fertility potential. It may also reduce the neurologic symptoms secondary to adenoma, especially if the growth is larger than 1 centimeter, extends outside the sella turcica (the bony structure in the skull encasing the pituitary), and presses on the optic nerve or the cavernous or sphenoid sinuses (air cavities in the cranial bones).

In my practice, I have observed a large number of patients with hyperprolactinemia and normal serum testosterone regain sexual desire following treatment with one of the preceding medications. Furthermore, even some patients with normal serum prolactin and testosterone have responded to the medications for unknown reasons, which may include a direct effect on the brain centers responsible for desire. Further controlled, multi-institutional, double-blind, prospective studies are warranted to confirm these initial observations.

The side effects of these drugs include nausea, postural hypotension (drop of blood pressure on standing up), and mental fogginess. Other less common reactions are depression, alcohol intolerance, stuffy nose, and Raynaud's phenomenon, which is marked vasoconstriction of the hands' peripheral arteries on exposure to cold. In some cases, if there is no response to pharmacotherapy or if the adenoma is more than 3 centimeters in size, surgical excision may be indicated. Radiation therapy is used primarily to prevent recurrence after excision of a giant tumor. (For women, in cases of pregnancy with hyperprolactinemia or following treatment, bromocriptine can be administered throughout the pregnancy without endangering the fetus.)

Hypogonadism

Hypogonadism is a condition resulting from a lower than normal level of testosterone. Total serum testosterone is composed of three portions: one is free (unbound) testosterone, one is loosely bound to the protein albumin, and one is bound to serum hormone-binding globulin (SHBG). Only the free and albumin-bound portions are biologically active or bioavailable to modulate the androgen functions described previously. SHBG, which is inactive, slowly releases its bound testosterone portion into the circulation as free or albumin-bound testosterone. About 2% of a normal male's serum testosterone is free, about 65% is bound to albumin, and the rest is bound to SHBG. In adulthood, any excessive decline in serum testosterone concentration, especially free testosterone, may cause sexual dysfunctions, including partial or complete loss of libido.

Concentrations of SHBG vary from person to person and change due to age or chronic disease, affecting testosterone measurement. The numerous conditions that can skew measured testosterone values by lowering or raising SHBG include aging, obesity, hypothyroidism, the metabolic syndrome, administration of male or female hormones, nephrotic syndrome (degenerative kidney disease with edema, high serum cholesterol, and increased excretion of albumin in the urine), acromegaly (hypersecretion of pituitary growth hormone with enlargement of the bones), aging, hyperthyroidism, HIV infection, liver cirrhosis, and using anticonvulsants. Therefore accurate measurements of active (i.e., free and albumin-bound) testosterone are essential for the diagnosis and treatment of hypogonadism.

As a man ages, his serum testosterone naturally declines approximately 1% per year after age 50. However, the rate of decrease is not constant: about 2% to 5% for ages 40–49, 6% to 30% for ages 50–59, 20% to 45% for ages 60–69, 43% to 70% for ages 70–79, and 91% over the age of 80. When testosterone decreases in older men and clinical changes occur, some physicians attribute these changes to aging in general and others to testosterone decline specifically. Decreased concentration of this hormone with age, accompanied by its clinical symptoms, has been given various names such as andropause, androgen decline in the aging male, and symptomatic late onset hypogonadism. In contrast to menopause, its onset is slow and insidious (Sultan C et al. 2001, Montorsi F et al. 2003, Kratzik CW et al. 2004, Schubert M, Jockenhovel F 2005).

It has been estimated from the Massachusetts Male Aging Study (MMAS) following 1,576 men for eight years that approximately 2.5 million men aged 40–69 suffer from hypogonadism in the United States—that is, a prevalence of about 12.3% per 100,000 men—with about 481,000 new cases per year (Araujo AB et al. 2004). The nonspecific signs and symptoms of androgen deficiency include the following:

Diminished sexual desire
Poor nocturnal erections during sleep
ED or sex-induced erections (controversial) (Vignozzi L et al. 2005)
Decreased intellectual abilities, memory loss, reduced mental concentration
Disturbed spatial orientation
Changes in mood
Depression, grumpiness, sadness, anger, and/or decreased enjoyment of life
Diminished muscle mass, strength, energy, endurance, and/or ability to exercise
Decreased motivation, initiative, self-confidence, and aggressiveness
Insomnia and sleep disturbances, sleepiness after meals, fatigue
Deteriorated work performance
Accumulation of fat in the lower abdomen
Decreased body hair and body height, slow beard growth

Anemia, skin alterations, muscle aches, possible osteoporosis
Increased incidence of hip fractures, type 2 diabetes, and low high-density lipoprotein (HDL, "good" cholesterol)

Testosterone deficiency syndrome is associated with a twofold increase in cardiovascular and overall mortality as well as a 3.3-fold increase in cancer-related mortality, as reported by the Massachusetts Longitudinal Aging Study (Araujo AB et al. 2004).

Hypogonadism is associated with an increased risk of diabetes and coronary artery disease.

Although hypogonadism has been correlated with an increased incidence of prostate cancer as well as with a worse grade and stage of the cancer, the MMAS found no correlation of prostate cancer with levels of total serum testosterone, free testosterone, SHBG, estradiol, or androstenedione (Morales A 2006).

With the occurrence of some of the preceding symptoms, and especially when at least two successive laboratory evaluations performed between 8:00 A.M. and 10:00 A.M. demonstrate a serum testosterone level below the normal value of 200 or 300 micrograms per deciliter or a definitive decline in the free or bioavailable testosterone, the diagnosis of androgen deficiency can be made with confidence.

Treatment of hypogonadism with testosterone should be reserved for men with documented low serum testosterone and significant signs and symptoms of the deficiency. Recent application of structured inventories, such as the ANDROTEST, may assist physicians in diagnosing hypogonadism in men with ED and in applying an appropriate and adequate therapy (Morelli A et al. 2007). Administration can be via gel, skin patches, a buccal system (tablets placed on the gums), intramuscular injections, subcutaneous pellets, or oral testosterone. The characteristics of the different forms of testosterone replacement therapy (TRT) are illustrated in Table 16.1. They may boost sexual desire and may improve sexual functioning. They may also improve mental abilities, mood, muscle strength, concentration, bone mass, vigor, and physical performance as well as countering anemia, reducing the incidence of osteoporosis-related fractures, increasing well-being and quality of life, and decreasing cardiovascular risk and death. A recent study comparing the long-term effect of testosterone gel and undecanoate injections on sexual dysfunction and the metabolic syndrome confirmed their beneficial effect, with an advantage for the injections in raising and maintaining a normal level of serum testosterone (Saad F et al. 2008). TRT should be individualized to obtain optimal results with minimal side effects, and patients should be monitored periodically to assess its effectiveness and watch for adverse reactions.

Table 16.1
Characteristics of Various Forms of Testosterone (T) Replacement Therapy

Route of administration	Drug	Special characteristics	Side effects and disadvantages
Oral	Methyltesterone Fluoxymesterone	Variable and low bioavailability	Potential liver toxicity No longer used in the USA
	Testosterone Testosteroneundecanoate (lipisoluble)	May produce physiologic serum levels of testosterone (T) Optimal absorption if ingested during fatty meals	Variable absorption and serum testosterone levels May block pituitary testicular axis and cause infertility
	Mesterolone	No effect on pituitary testicular axis Used for the treatment of male infertility Variable bioavailability and serum testosterone levels	Not available in the United States Not available in the United States

Intramuscular injections	Testosterone cypionate	Administered in fixed doses every two to three weeks	Supra- and infraphysiologic concentrations of serum testosterone with no diurnal variation
	Testosterone enanthate (200–250 mg)	Long-acting effect	
		Rapid action and steady decline	May cause male infertility and absence of sperms in the semen
			Painful intramuscular injections every two to three weeks
			Higher incidence of increased number of red blood cells
	Testosterone undecanoate 1000 mg	Long-acting effect (6–12 weeks)	Not available in the United States
		Repeated injections every 6–12 weeks	Slight increase in red blood cells
		Physiologic serum levels of testosterone	Pain at injection site possible
		No supraphysiologic variations	May cause male infertility
Skin patches (Scrotal and unscrotal)	Testosterone patches of 2.5–5 mg (applied at night)	Replicates normal diurnal rhythm of testosterone secretion	May cause skin irritation and sensitization

(continued)

Table 16.1 (*continued*)

Route of administration	Drug	Special characteristics	Side effects and disadvantages
		Physiologic testosterone serum levels	May not achieve normal testosterone serum concentrations
		Few office visits	Possible lack of skin adhesion, especially in scrotum
			May cause male infertility
			Scrotal patches require shaving
			Expensive (about $100/month)
Skin gel	5–7.5 g of gel daily applied in the morning on specific areas of the skin (shoulders, upper arms, and lower abdomen)	Most popular form of treatment	Possible drug accumulation
		Normal serum levels of testosterone over 24 hours	Possible variability in serum levels of testosterone
		Odorless and nonmessy	
		Easy to use, with high patient compliance	May cause male infertility
			Expensive (about $170/month)
			May be transferred through skin contact to children or women

Oral (gums) tablets (SUTENT)	30 g tablets adherent to gums twice daily	Physiologic levels of testosterone	May cause gum irritation and possible bad breath
		Good and rapid absorption through gums	Very expensive (about $200/month)
		No hepatotoxicity	
			Twice daily application
			May not stick to gums
		Effect may last several months	May cause infertility
Subcutaneous implantation	Testosterone pellets under the skin		Requires skin incision
		Variability in testosterone serum levels	
			Variable serum levels of testosterone
		Does not replicate physiological diurnal in the testosterone	May cause infertility

NEWSFLASH: PARTICULAR BENEFITS OF TESTOSTERONE THERAPY IN SOME CASES OF HYPOGONADISM AND SEXUAL DYSFUNCTION

Recently, hypogonadism has been associated with an unhealthy condition called metabolic syndrome. This syndrome is characterized by central obesity, insulin resistance with type 2 diabetes or impaired glucose tolerance, increased serum triglycerides (neutral fats synthesized from carbohydrates), decreased concentration of the good cholesterol called high density lipoproteins (HDL), and hypertension. Testosterone therapy can slow or avert metabolic syndrome's progression toward overt diabetes and cardiovascular disease and can prevent the occurrence of associated sexual dysfunction, especially in cases with a marked decline in free testosterone. Hypogonadism and erectile dysfunction both appear to be more common among men infected with HIV, who may also respond well to testosterone replacement therapy.

Testosterone replacement is contraindicated in the presence of prostate or breast cancer, hardness or nodule(s) or asymmetry in the prostate, serum prostate-specific antigen level over 3 micrograms per milliliter, hematocrit (volume of red blood cells in centrifuged blood sample) over 50%, untreated sleep apnea, severe heart failure, or severe lower urinary tract symptoms due to benign prostatic hyperplasia. Possible side effects include a possible stimulation of occult (hidden) prostate cancer, although recent studies failed to reveal an increased incidence of this tumor with testosterone administration (Gaylis FD et al. 2005), unproven increased prostatic volume with worsened urinary symptoms, fluid retention, gynecomastia (growth of the male's breasts), decreased level of HDL (the good) cholesterol the and polycythemia (increased red cell mass in the blood). Of particular concern is the development or worsening of sleep apnea, which is characterized by significant snoring, daytime sleepiness, and periods of arrested breathing for about 20 seconds or more during sleep, which rarely can be fatal and which require prompt diagnosis and management, with the discontinuation of the testosterone therapy. Other complications with some oral testosterone preparations—not approved or available in the United States—may be decreased HDL and possible liver toxicity.

OTHER MAJOR ETIOLOGIES

Aside from hormonal issues, several additional biological and psychological factors may contribute to decreased sexual desire. Aging, various medical conditions, eating disorders, antidepressant medications, and bodybuilding are the most common. Other causes of low libido include depression, anxiety, anger, posttraumatic stress syndrome, and relationship conflict (Meuleman EJH, Van Lankveld JDM 2004).

Aging

Aging is probably the most common physical cause of hypoactive sexual desire, with a gradual decline in libido typically experienced after age 40 (Rosen RC 2005). This does not mean, however, that older men or women are not interested in sex. Quite the contrary: almost two-thirds maintain a mild to moderate desire to engage in sexual activity. Although various chronic medical conditions and medications may temper this urge, the majority of older men may nevertheless develop good erections, albeit softer than before, and can reach climax and ejaculate satisfactorily. Some elderly men experience depression, anxiety, absence of a partner, fear of death, and familial and psychological problems, any of which could hamper their sexual desire. But in the absence of hypogonadism, testosterone treatment is not indicated.

Medical Conditions

Medical causes for loss of sexual desire include stroke, epilepsy, hypothyroidism, chronic renal failure, CAD, heart failure, HIV infection/AIDS, and chronic arthritis. Patients on dialysis for kidney disease are more often affected by low libido than those who have received a renal transplant. Medications such as female hormones; GnRH; antiandrogens used for metastatic prostate cancer; and dopaminergic (dopamine-simulating) drugs, such as levodopa, used for Parkinson's disease, can lead to diminished desire as well. Unfortunately, no effective treatment for low libido stemming from most of these physical factors yet exists, short of changing or discontinuing medications— under medical supervision—if it is medically feasible, or replacing the thyroid hormone.

Psychiatric and Psychological Factors

Hypoactive desire is the most common sexual dysfunction in psychiatric outpatients, especially those with schizophrenia and taking neuroleptic medications or those with major depression (with or without medication). Low sexual desire may affect more than 40% of depressed men; on the other hand, about 10% may exhibit increased desire. Antidepressant medications can also lead to low libido, so depressed patients who are still interested in sex should use them carefully and selectively.

Relationship disturbances play a significant but often underestimated role in lessened sexual desire. Physical repulsion, hygiene issues, resentment, anger, suspicion, hatred, premature ejaculation, past traumatic sexual experiences, adultery, jealousy, and dissatisfaction with the relationship are important factors that may require psychotherapy and relationship/marriage counseling for their management.

THERAPIES ON THE HORIZON

Some recently investigated agents, such as androgen receptor modulators, which increase the effectiveness of testosterone receptors, may offer new avenues of safe and effective therapy for hypogonadism. Several pharmacologic agents, such as yohimbine, Nitromed (a combination of a nitric oxide donor, L-arginine, and yohimbine), and dopamine agonists, including high-dose sublingual apomorphine (Uprima; see chapter 11), have been introduced as potential stimulants of sexual desire. Like the androgen receptor modulators, they have yielded some encouraging preliminary results, but most of those studies lacked validated scoring systems and objective criteria to assess the compounds' efficacy and safety. Several pharmaceutical companies are now developing subtype-selective neuropeptide-Y antagonists that block the action of certain desire-lowering neurotransmitters, which may eventually prove useful for the management of low libido.

Some smells perceived at the conscious level, such as perfumes, may have the capability of inducing sexual desire in humans, possibly by enhancing other sensory cues, such as vision and touch, and contributing to a composite picture of an attractive partner (Goldmeier D, Green PE 1998). Pheromones, which are certain chemicals with odors that are perceived at the subliminal level, have been demonstrated to induce sexual desire, copulation, and reproduction in rhesus monkeys and pigs but have yet to prove their efficacy in humans.

A few recent studies, however, have suggested that some synthetic pheromones may increase the rates of men's sexual encounters and behavior. Another showed that adding a particular pheromone (of as yet unknown composition) to a man's shaving cream daily seems to increase his female partner's sexual desire (Cutler WB et al. 1998). The use of these substances may have great impact on the future management of low sexual desire, especially when combined with other modes of therapy, and warrants further study.

GLOSSARY

Please refer to this glossary to explain any unknown terms you may encounter in this book. Many doctors erroneously expect their routine medical terminology to be easily understood, but to readers, medical jargon often seems like a foreign language.

Abstinence: Refraining from sexual intercourse.

Androgens: The group of male sex hormones that promote masculinization. Beginning at puberty, they stimulate development of the male external and internal genital organs, growth of body hair, changes in the voice, and growth of muscle and bone. They may also initiate sexual desire and activities.

Arteriosclerosis: An abnormal thickening and loss of elasticity of the arterial walls in any part of the body. A significant cause of organic erectile dysfunction and cardiovascular disease.

Atherosclerosis: The clogging of the arteries by plaques containing cholesterol, fatlike material, fat-containing cells, and platelets.

Autonomic Nerves: Those nerves that function without voluntary or conscious control. Also called the self-governing or involuntary nervous system. Includes the parasympathetic and sympathetic nerves, which are responsible for the activity of cardiac muscle, smooth muscle, and internal genital organs as well as emission and ejaculation of semen and secretions of various glands. *See also* Nervous System.

Autonomic Nervous System: A subsystem of the nervous system; a portion of both the central and peripheral nervous systems, over which there is no voluntary or conscious control. The autonomic nervous system is further divided into the sympathetic nervous system and the parasympathetic nervous system, each of which has a different effect on organs such as the heart, intestines, stomach, and the internal genitalia. Both systems are involved in erection, emission, and ejaculation.

Blood Sinuses: Vascular spaces that fill with blood.

Central Nervous System: The central nervous system is located in the cranium (skull) and the spine. The brain and the spinal cord connect through an opening in the base of the skull to form a continuous central system. A human being has 12 pairs of cranial nerves, which are connected to the brain, and 31 pairs of spinal nerves, which are associated with the spinal cord.

Chordee: A curvature or unusual bending of the erect penis due to various congenital or acquired causes. *See also* Peyronie's Disease.

Climax: The peak sexual sensation and gratification of the sexual act. The culmination of orgasm and ejaculation.

Corpora Cavernosa: Two spongy tissue channels, one on each side of the penis, in the shape of sausages, containing blood vessels and vascular spaces laid on a frame of fibro-elastic tissue and smooth muscles, which run from the glans penis (head) back into the body. When the penis is flaccid, about 40% to 50% of these corpora are in the portion of the shaft outside the body; in the erect penis, that amount increases to about 60% to 70% of the corpora. The sacral nerves control the flow of blood into the compartments of the corpora cavernosa, which must fill with blood for the penis to become erect.

Corpus Spongiosum: Spongy tissue surrounding the urethra in the penis. Does not play a role in the erectile process other than engorgement.

Cowper's Glands: Paired pea-sized glands located below the prostate that drain directly into the urethra. They produce the clear drops of fluid, often called "nature's lubrication" or "precum," that appear at the meatus (opening) of the urethra in the glans penis during sexual arousal. They contribute to the washing of urine from the urethra and to its lubrication during sexual arousal and prior to sexual intercourse. These drops may contain live sperms.

Diabetes Mellitus: A chronic disease caused either by insufficient production of insulin by the pancreas (type 1) or by the body's resistance to insulin (type 2). When advanced, it can cause erectile dysfunction as a result of damage done to the blood vessels and nerves leading to and within the penis.

Diagnosis: The method applied for determining the nature of a disease or disorder and its underlying cause(s).

Diplomate: A title indicating a physician who is board certified in his or her specialty.

Ejaculation: The emission of semen through the urinary channel to the outside of the penis during orgasm.

Ejaculatory Ducts: The small tubes that traverse the prostate gland and connect the seminal vesicles and the vasa deferentia to the urethra. Carry part of the semen and sperms into the urethra during climax and ejaculation.

Endocrine System: The various glands (the pituitary, thyroid, parathyroid, pancreas, and adrenal glands as well as the testicles and ovaries) that secrete hormones into the bloodstream, affecting and controlling the function of various organs.

The pituitary gland is the so-called master gland of the endocrine system, with its secretion of essential hormones that regulate the function of various glands such as the thyroid, the adrenal glands, and the testicles. It also secretes the hormone prolactin (essential for lactation).

The thyroid gland's secretion of the hormone thyroxin regulates the body's metabolism. Hypo- or hypersecretion by this gland may produce erectile dysfunction.

The parathyroid gland, via parathyroid hormone, controls the blood's concentration of calcium and phosphate.

The pancreas secretes the hormone insulin, which permits the body's cells to metabolize and utilize sugar.

The adrenal gland is basically composed of two independent parts. The cortex (outer part) contains hormones (mainly cortisone) that play a pivotal role in body homeostasis such as, among other things, maintaining resistance to physical and emotional stress; balancing the levels of electrolytes, minerals, and some sex hormones in the bloodstream; and playing a primary role in blood pressure control. The medulla (inner part) manufactures the hormone adrenaline (epinephrine), which stimulates the circulatory system and sympathetic nervous system (constricting blood vessels and raising blood pressure).

The testicles produce sperms and testosterone, the male hormone that controls development of male secondary sexual characteristics, male libido (sex drive), and male sexual functioning.

The ovaries produce the ova and secrete the female hormones.

Endocrinology: The branch of medical science that specializes in the diagnosis and treatment of diseases and disorders of the endocrine system and its hormones.

Engorgement: Being filled with blood.

Epilepsy: A brain disorder characterized by the presence of seizures, which is caused by many different underlying conditions. Can be a primary cause of erectile dysfunction.

Erectile Dysfunction (or Impotence): The inability of a man to achieve or maintain an erection for a period long enough for satisfactory intercourse. *See also* Sexual Dysfunction.

Erection: The enlargement and rigidity of the upstanding penis when it becomes engorged (filled with blood). A normal erection depends on the integrity of the neurovascular system and the male hormone system.

Etiology: Refers to the causes of a disease, condition, or disorder. The term *etiology* is also used in medical slang as a synonym for causes.

External Vacuum Device: A plastic cylinder with a suction device, applied over the penis to create a vacuum around the penis. When the suction produces an erection, a plastic or rubber ring is applied at the base of the penis to maintain the erection.

FACS (Fellow of the American College of Surgeons): Signifying a physician's qualification as a surgical specialist and as a member of this association.

Fibrosis: The replacement of the normal tissue of an organ or other body structure with fibrous growth, for example, scarring.

Flaccidity: The normally lax, soft, nonerect state of the penis.

Frenulum: The skin fold located on the lower part of the glans penis, connecting it to the prepuce.

Ganglia: Groups of nerve cell bodies located outside the central nervous system, for example, in the pelvis or alongside the spinal cord, and interconnected with nerves.

Glans Penis: The sensitive, gland-shaped head of the penis, located at the distal end and covered by the prepuce.

Hormone: A chemical substance, produced in the body by the cells of a gland, that regulates various bodily functions and processes such as growth, reproduction, and metabolism. Hormones affecting sexual function are principally produced in the pituitary gland, adrenal glands, testicles, and ovaries. *See also* Endocrine System.

Hypogonadism: A decrease in the serum concentration of testosterone because of its inadequate secretion by the testicles due to lesions affecting them or the pituitary gland.

Hypospadias: An abnormal location of the urethral meatus at the lower part of the glans penis, on the penile shaft, at the junction of the penis and the scrotum or in the scrotum or perineum.

Libido: Sexual desire or sex drive. It is initiated in the sex centers of the brain under the influence of sensual, emotional, or sexual stimuli or fantasies. It usually requires a normal concentration of serum testosterone, especially in men.

Ligation: The surgical procedure that consists in tying off a blood vessel or other tube that may be applied to abnormal leaking penile veins as a means of slowing the outflow (or leakage) of blood from the penis to achieve and/or maintain erection.

Microphallus (or Micropenis): A penis that is abnormally small according to well-established medical norms and standards.

Muscles (as Related to the Erection Process): Specialized tissues capable of movement by contracting and relaxing, and thereby contributing to numerous bodily activities and functions.

> The bulbo cavernosum muscles surround the corpora cavernosa and contract during ejaculation to expel semen outside the body.
> The bulbo spongiosum muscle envelops the corpus spongiosum and protects the urethra.
> The cremaster muscle pulls the testicles up toward the abdomen or allows them to droop or sag in the scrotum. This, among other things, acts as a temperature regulator for sperms.
> The dartos muscle tightens the skin of the scrotum.
> Vascular smooth muscles, located within the blood vessels throughout the body and in the penile arteries, dilate or constrict the vessels, thereby regulating blood flow into and out of the penis.

Nervous System (as Related to the Erectile Process): A network of neurons, neurochemicals, and other related structures that function to receive sensory stimuli, generate responses, and control bodily activities. The nervous system is composed essentially of two separate but interrelated parts: the central nervous system and the peripheral nervous system. *See also* Central Nervous System; Autonomic Nervous System; Peripheral Nervous System.

Neurology: A medical specialty in the diagnosis and treatment of neurological diseases.

Orgasm: The sudden and intense sexual pleasure experienced by the male prior to ejaculation and by the female during climax that is perceived in the brain. It represents the culmination of sexual excitement and gratification.

Penile Prosthesis: A manufactured semirigid or inflatable device surgically implanted within the corpora cavernosa of the penis, enabling a man to have an erectionlike state on demand and to maintain it for as long as desired.

Penis: The male sex organ. Provides a conduit for the passage of urine, the means to have sexual intercourse, and a conduit for the transport and deposit of semen.

Perineum: The area between the anus and the scrotum.

Peripheral (or Distal): Near the surface, distant, the opposite of proximal. The glans, for example, is the distal end of the penis.

Peripheral Nervous System: Peripheral nerves supply stimulation and sensation to the arms, legs, and other portions of the body distant from the central nervous system.

The cutaneous nerves supply sensation to the skin throughout the body.
The genitofemoral nerves supply skin sensation to the testicles and adjacent areas.
The ilioinguinal nerves and scrotal nerves supply sensation to the scrotum.
The pudendal nerves carry penile sensations through the spinal cord to the brain and are involved in contracting the bulbo cavernosum muscles during ejaculation.
The sacral nerves, which supply genitourinary organs such as the bladder and the penis, play a primary role in the erectile and ejaculatory processes and in voiding.

Peyronie's Disease: A penile curvature or bend resulting from a plaque (scar tissue or fibrosis) between the corpora cavernosa and the tunica albuginea (sheath around the penis). Can cause pain and abnormal angulation during an erection and sometimes erectile dysfunction. The resulting awkward shape ("the bent spike") can sometimes prevent intercourse. *See also* Chordee.

Phimosis: A tight foreskin over the head of the penis that cannot be retracted.

Physical or Organic Erectile (or Sexual) Dysfunction: Erectile (or sexual) dysfunction resulting from physical or organic disease(s) or disorder(s) as opposed to psychological reasons.

Plexus: A network of blood vessels or nerves.

Premature Ejaculation: The uncontrolled discharge of semen before the desired time, causing distress to the afflicted man or to the couple. Very common condition.

Priapism: An erection lasting an abnormally long time (four hours or more), unassociated with ongoing sexual pleasure. May be painful and could cause permanent damage to the penis such as fibrosis.

Prostate Gland: A walnut-shaped male gland located below the bladder neck. Secretes part of the seminal fluid that transports sperms during ejaculation, usually producing about 20% to 30% of the ejaculate volume.

Proximal: Near the center of the body, opposite peripheral or distal. The base of the penile shaft, for example, is the proximal end of the penis.

Psychogenic Erectile (or Sexual) Dysfunction: Erectile (or sexual) problem having a psychological rather than a physical etiology.

REM (Rapid Eye Movements): The stage of sleep in which dreams occur and which is characterized by rapid movements of the eyes. During REM sleep, most men have, according to their age, from one to six erections, which can last 10–20 minutes each. A doctor may evaluate nocturnal erections as part of diagnostic testing.

Revascularization: A surgical procedure rerouting the blood supply to an organ due to an obstructed or constricted artery supplying the organ. A viable, although rarely applied, treatment option in the few selected men for whom an arterial blood inflow or venous outflow problem is the cause of their erectile dysfunction.

Scrotum: In males, the external pocket of skin that envelops and contains the testicles.

Semen: The fluid, produced by the seminal vesicles, the prostate, and the testicles, that carries the sperms from the testicles and provides them with nutrients. Stored in either the vas deferens or its reservoir and ejaculated at orgasm.

Seminal Vesicles: A pair of pouches located in the pelvis, behind and lateral to the prostate. They secrete the major portion of the semen during climax, producing about 70% of the ejaculate volume.

Sensate Focus: A technique, used in sex therapy, of focusing on the sensual pleasure of foreplay.

Sexual Dysfunction: The broad spectrum of organic and/or psychogenic sexual disorders in males and females. In males, often called "erectile dysfunction" or "impotence."

Sexually Functional: Able to perform sexual activities satisfactorily.

Sleep Laboratory: A doctor's office, clinic, or laboratory in which testing for erections occurring during sleep may be carried out.

Sperm: The male reproductive cell, which carries a set of the male's genes and is usually capable of fertilizing the female ovum (egg). Manufactured in the testicles and emitted from the body in semen through the penis.

Spinal Column: The flexible chain of bones, disks, and ligaments that encases the spinal cord. Composed of four portions:

The cervical spine in the neck contains the first seven vertebrae.
The thoracic (or dorsal) spine immediately below the neck in the upper back contains 12 thoracic vertebrae.
The lumbar spine in the lower back contains five lumbar vertebrae.
The sacrococcygeal spine in the posterior wall of the pelvis contains five fused (joined) sacral vertebrae and four fused coccygeal vertebrae.

Spinal Cord: An extension of the brain, encased in protective membranes and containing 31 pairs of spinal nerves distributed evenly down the entire length of the spinal column. It acts as a conduit or a pathway between the brain and the rest of the body, collecting sensory information from the body and sending nervous messages from the brain for proper functioning of various organs.

Suprapubic Fat Pad: A large mass of fat over the suprapubic area.

Testicles: A pair of walnut-sized male organs enclosed in the scrotum. The testicles produce sperms and testosterone. Testicle size in adults varies from male to male. The left testicle is usually lower than the right testicle, and one can be larger than the other. The testicles' ascent and descent into and out of the scrotum is a reflex action of the cremaster muscles, which surround the spermatic cords. The testicles produce less than 1% of the ejaculate volume.

Testosterone: The principal male hormone, produced and secreted mainly by the testicles. Among other things, it stimulates the development of male secondary sexual characteristics during puberty, including the penis and the masculine contours of the adult male body. Also involved in sexual functioning, fertility, and sexual desire, and may have an impact on the normal function of various other organs.

Tumescence: An elongation and swelling. The beginning state of an erection, during which the penis is expanding but not yet hard. *See also* Engorgement.

Urethra: The urinary channel. In men, it extends from the neck of the bladder to the external meatus at the tip of the glans penis. In women, it extends from the neck of the bladder to its external opening below the clitoris at the roof of the vaginal outlet.

Urology: The surgical specialty in the diagnosis and medical and surgical treatment of genitourinary diseases, male infertility, and sexual disorders.

Vacuum Erection Device: A mechanical device, normally consisting of a penile cylinder, pump (piston or pneumatic), and penile rings, used by a man to obtain and maintain an erection.

Vas Deferens: The tube that carries sperms from the testicle to the urethra. (The plural is *vasa deferentia*.) Sperms are stored in the vas deferens and its ampulla (reservoir) preparatory to ejaculation.

Vascular System (as Related to Erection): The body's network of blood vessels, including arteries, veins, and capillaries. In erection, arteries carry blood from the heart to the penis, and veins carry blood from the penis to the heart. Names of blood vessels are usually derived from the part of the body in which they are found, or from the organ that they supply.

The cavernosal artery supplies blood to the corpus cavernosum of the penis.
The internal iliac artery supplies some pelvic organs and the genitalia, including the bladder, prostate, seminal vesicles, and penis.
The penile dorsal artery supplies blood to the top skin of the penis and to the glans penis.
The testicular (or spermatic) arteries supply the testicles.

Vasoconstriction: The contraction and narrowing of blood vessels. A cause of erectile dysfunction.

Vasodilator: A chemical substance that causes the opening, widening, and expansion of the blood vessels and blood spaces (vascular sinuses filled with blood).

BIBLIOGRAPHY

Althof SE, et al. "Why do so many people drop out from auto-injection therapy for impotence?" *J Sex Marital Ther* 15:121–129, 1989.

Althof SE, et al. "Psychological and interpersonal dimensions of sexual function and dysfunction." Paper presented at the Second International Consultation on Erectile and Sexual Dysfunctions. Paris, June 28–July 1, 2003.

Althof SE, et al. "Psychological and interpersonal dimensions of sexual function and dysfunction." *J Dex Med* 2:793–800, 2005.

American Psychiatric Association. *Diagnostic and Statistical Manual of Mental Disorders.* 4th ed. Washington, DC: American Psychiatric Press, 1994.

Althof SE, et al. "Psychological and interpersonal dimensions of sexual function and dysfunction." *J Dex Med* 2:793–800, 2005.

Araujo AB, et al. "Changes in sexual function in middle-aged and older men: longitudinal data from the Massachusetts Male Aging Study." *J Am Geriatr Soc* 52:1502–1509, 2004.

Austoni E, et al. "A new technique for augmentation phalloplasty: albugineal surgery with bilateral saphenous grafts: three years of experience." *Eur Urol* 42:345–353, 2002.

Awwad Z, et al. "Penile measurements in normal adult Jordanians and in patients with erectile dysfunction." *Int J Impot Res* 17:191–195, 2005.

Bannowsky A, et al. "Recovery of erectile function after nerve sparing prostatectomy—improvement with nightly low dose sildenafil." Paper presented at the American Urological Association Annual Meeting. Atlanta, GA, May 20–25, 2006.

Bansal TC, et al. "Incidence of metabolic syndrome and insulin resistance in a population with organic erectile dysfunction." *J Sex Med* 2:96–103, 2005.

Barada J, McCullough AR. "Premature ejaculation: increasing recognition and improving treatment." *MD Medscape Today,* June 2, 2004, htt://bcbsma.medscape.com/viewprogram/3131.

Basson R, et al. [No title]. Paper presented at the Second International Consultation on Erectile and Sexual Dysfunctions. Paris, June 28–July 1, 2003.

Bayer-Glaxo Co. "Vardenafil hydrochloride (Levitra)." U.S. prescribing information, 2003.

Becker AJ, et al. "Therapy of organic erectile dysfunction" (in German). *Urologe A* 44: 1160–1166, 2005.

Beheri GE, "Surgical treatment of impotence." *Plas. Reconst Surgery* 38:92–97, 1966.

Bella AJ, et al. "Non-palpable scarring of the penile septum as a cause of ED: an atypical form of Peyronie's disease." Paper presented at the American Urological Association Annual Meeting. Atlanta, GA, May 20–25, 2006.

Bennett AH. "Revascularization using the dorsal vein of the penis in vasculogenic impotence." *Semin Urol* 4:259–262, 1986.

Benson CB, Vickers MA. "Sexual impotence caused by vascular disease: diagnosis with duplex sonography." *Am J Roenthenol* 153:1149–1153, 1989.

Blanker MH, et al. "Correlates for erectile and ejaculatory dysfunction in older Dutch men: a community-based study." *J Am Geriatr Soc* 49:436–442, 2001.

Blundell N. *The World's Greatest Scandals of the Twentieth Century.* London: Hamlyn/Reed Octopus Publishing Gray Ltd., pp. 137–139, 1994.

Bondil P, et al. "Educational, socio-cultural and ethical aspects of sexual dysfunction." Paper presented at the Second International Consultation on Erectile and Sexual Dysfunctions. Paris, June 28–July 1, 2003.

Bookstein JJ, et al. "Pharmacoangiographic assessment of the corpora cavernosa." *Cardiovasc Intervent Radiol* 11:218–224, 1988.

Brandstetter K, et al. "Color duplex sonography of the penis—examination technique and clinical results." *Bildgebung* 58:42–44, 1991.

Brant MD, et al. "The prosthesis salvage operation: immediate replacement of the infected penile prosthesis." *J Urol* 155:155–157, 1996.

Braun M, et al. "Epidemiology of erectile dysfunction: results of the 'Cologne Male Survey.'" *Int J Impot Res* 12:305–311, 2000.

Brinkman MJ, et al. "A survey of patients with inflatable penile prostheses for satisfaction." *J Urol* 174:352–357, 2005.

Brissard E. "How to become a multiorgasmic man?" (in French). *Psychologies* 8:55, 2006.

Brisson TE, et al. "Vardenafil rescue rates of sildenafil nonresponders: objective assessment of 327 patients with erectile dysfunction." *Urology* 68:397–401, 2006.

Broderick GA, et al. "The hemodynamics of vacuum constriction erections: assessment by color Doppler ultrasound. *J Urol* 147:57–61, 1992.

Cappelleri JC, Rosen RC. "The Sexual Health Inventory for Men (SHIM): a 5-year review of research and clinical experience." *Int J Impot Res* 17:307–319, 2005.

Carson CC, Lue TF. "Phosphodiesterase type 5 inhibitors for erectile dysfunction." *BJU Int* 96:257–268, 2005.

Carson CC, et al. "The 'effectiveness' scale—therapeutic outcome of pharmacologic therapies for ED: an international consensus panel report." *Int J Impot* 16:207–213, 2004.

Carson CC, et al. "Erectile dysfunction: new concepts in diagnosis, prevention, and management." Paper presented at the American Urological Association Annual Meeting. Atlanta, GA, May 20–25, 2006.

Cavallini G, et al. "Oral propionyl-1-carnitine and intraplaque verapamil in the therapy of advanced and resistant Peyronie's disease." *BJU Int* 89:895–900, 2002.

Chen J, et al. "Predicting penile size during erection." *Int J Impot Res* 12:328–333, 2000.

Chen KL, et al. "Total corpora replacement for erectile dysfunction." Paper presented at the American Urological Association Annual Meeting. Atlanta, GA, May 20–25, 2006.

Chia SJ, et al. "Clinical application of prognostic factor for patients with organic causes of erectile dysfunction on 100 mg of sildenafil citrate." *Int J Urol* 11:1104–1109, 2004.

Corona G, et al. "Aging and pathogenesis of erectile dysfunction." *Int J Impot Res* 16:395–402, 2004.

Cutler WB, et al. "Pheromonal influences in sociosexual behavior." *Arch Sex Behav* 27:113, 1998.

De Amicis LA, et al. "Clinical follow up of couples treated for sexual dysfunction." *Arch Sex Behav* 14:467–489, 1985.

Dean J, et al. "Is premature ejaculation all in the mind?" *Br J Urol* 96:234–236, 2005.

De Berardis G, et al. "Clinical and psychological predictors of self reported erectile dysfunction in patients with type 2 diabetes." *J Urol* 177:252–257, 2007.

De Boer BJ, et al. "The prevalence of bother, acceptance, and need for help in men with erectile dysfunction." *J Sex Med* 2:445–450, 2005.

De la Taille A, et al. "Reasons for drop-out from short and long-term self injection therapy for impotence." *Eur Urol* 35:312–317, 1995.

Diemer T, et al. "Therapy of the aging male" (in German). *Urologe A* 44:1173–1178, 2005.

Dorland's Illustrated M Dictionary. 28th ed. Philadelphia: W. B. Saunders, 1994.

Dunajska K, et al. "Evaluation of sex hormone levels and some metabolic factors in men with coronary atherosclerosis." *Aging Male* 7:197–204, 2004.

Eardley I. "Vardenafil: a new oral treatment for erectile dysfunction." *Int J Clin Pract* 58:801–806, 2004.

Eardley I. "A closer look at the PDE-5 inhibitors (course)." Paper presented at the European Association of Urology Meeting. Istanbul, Turkey, March 16–19, 2005.

Eardley I, et al. "An open-label, multicentre, randomized, crossover study comparing sildenafil citrate and tadalafil for treating erectile dysfunction in men naïve to phosphodiesterase-5 inhibitor therapy." *Br J Urol Int* 96:1323–1332, 2005.

Eardley I, et al. "Factors associated with preference for sildenafil citrate and tadalafil for treating erectile dysfunction in men naive to phosphodiesterase 5 inhibitor therapy: post hoc analysis of data from a multicentre, randomized, open label, crossover study." *Br J Urol Int* 100:122–129, 2007.

Ebstein RP. "Sexual desire is in your genes: Israeli research." *ScienceNewsDen.com*, 2006, http://www.sciencenewsden.com/2006/sexualdesireisinyourgenes.shtml.

Fallon B. "Intracavernous injection therapy for male erectile dysfunction." *Urol Clin North Am* 22:833–845, 1995.

Fantini GV, et al. "Microvascular arterial bypass surgery: assessment of long-term outcome." Paper presented at the American Urological Association Annual Meeting. Atlanta, GA, May 20–25, 2006.

Feldman HA, et al. "Impotence and its medical and psychological correlates: results of the Massachusetts Male Aging Study." *J Urol* 151:54–61, 1994.

Frajese GV, Pozzi F. "New achievements and novel therapeutic applications of PDE-5 inhibitors in older males." *J Endocrinol Invest* 28:45–50, 2005.

Francken AB, et al. "What importance do women attribute to the size of the penis?" *Eur Urol* 42:426–431, 2002.

Furlow WL, Fisher J, Knoll LD, et al. "Current status of penile revascularization with deep dorsal vein arterialization. Experience with 95 patients." *Int J Impotence Res* 2:348–349, 1990.

Gallo L, et al. "Recovery of erection after pelvic urologic surgery: our experience." *Int J Impot Res* 17:45–48, 2005.

Gaylis FD, et al. "Prostate cancer in men using testosterone supplementation." *J Urol* 174:534–538, 2005.

Gelbard MK, et al. "The natural history of Peyronie's disease." *J Urol* 144:1376–1379, 1990.

Gemery JM, et al. "3D digital modeling of male pelvis on bicycle seats: impact of rider position and seat design on potential hypoxia and ED." Paper presented at the American Urological Association Annual Meeting. Atlanta, GA, May 20–25, 2006.

Gerstenberg TC, et al. "Intracavernous self-injection with vasoactive intestinal polypeptide and phentolamine in the management of erectile failure." *J Urol* 147:1277–1279, 1992.

Gholami SS, et al. "The effect of vascular endothelial growth factor and adeno-associated virus-mediated brain-derived neurotrophic factor on neurogenic and vasculogenic erectile dysfunction induced by hyperlipidemia." *J Urol* 169:1577–1581, 2003.

Goldmeier D, Green PE. "Pheromones = the smell of sexual desire." *Sex Dysfunc* 1:119–121, 1998.

Greenfield JM, et al. "Verapamil versus saline in electromotive drug administration (EDMA) for Peyronie's disease: a double blind controlled trial." Paper presented at the American Urological Association Annual Meeting. Atlanta, GA, May 20–25, 2006.

Gutierrez P, et al. "Combining programmed intracavernous PGE1 injections and sildenafil on demand to salvage sildenafil nonresponders." *Int J Impot Res* 17:354–358, 2005.

Hanash KA. "Comparative results of goal-oriented therapy for erectile dysfunction." *J Urol* 157:2135–2139, 1997.

Hanash KA, et al. *Perfect Lover: A Guide for Enhancing Everyone's Sex Life.* New York: SPI Books, 1994.

Harding R, Colombok SE. "Test-retest reliability of the measurement of penile dimensions in a sample of gay men." *Arch Sex Behav* 31:351–357, 2002.

Hatzichristou D, et al. "Effect of tadalafil on sexual timing behavior patterns in men with ED: integrated analysis of randomized placebo controlled trials." *J Urol* 174: 1356–1359, 2005.

Hatzimouratidis K, Hatzichristou DG. "A comparative review of the options for treatment of erectile dysfunction: which treatment for which patient?" *Drugs* 65:1621–1650, 2005.

Hatzimouratidis K, Hatzichristou DG. "Looking to the future for erectile dysfunction therapies." *Drugs* 68:231–250, 2008.

Havelock E. *Little Essays of Love and Virtue.* London: A & C Black, 1922.

Hellstrom WJG, et al. "Current safety and tolerability issues in men with erectile dysfunction receiving PDE-5 inhibitors." *Int J Clin Pract* 61:1547–1554, 2007.

Henry GD, et al. "Revision washout decreases penile prosthesis infection in revision surgery: a multicenter study." *J Urol* 173:89–92, 2005.

Herwig R, et al. "Pelvic venoablation with air-block aetoxysclerol for the treatment of erectile dysfunction caused by venous leakage." Paper presented at the American Urological Association Annual Meeting. Atlanta, GA, May 20–25, 2006.

Hutter AM, Jr. "Role of the cardiologist: clinical aspects of managing erectile dysfunction." *Clin Cardiol* 27:13–17, 2004.

Israilov S, et al. "Evaluation of a progressive treatment program for erectile dysfunction in patients with diabetes mellitus." *Int J Impot Res* 17:431–436, 2005.

Jannsen E, et al. "Automatic process and the appraisal of sexual stimuli: toward an information-processing model of sexual arousal." *J Sex Res* 37:8–23, 2000.

Jarrow JP, et al. "Course on male sexual dysfunction: practice management guidelines." Paper presented at the American Urological Association Annual Meeting. Atlanta, GA, May 20–25, 2006.

Johannes CB, et al. "Incidence of erectile dysfunction in men 40 to 69 years old: prospective results from the Massachusetts Male Aging Study." *J Urol* 163:460–463, 2000.

Kaiser FE, Korenman SG. "Erectile dysfunction in diabetic men." *JAMA* 85(suppl 5A):147–150, 1988.

Kalmuss D. "Nonvolitional sex and sexual health." *Arch Sex Behav* 33:197–209, 2004.

Kawanishi Y, et al. "Penile revascularization surgery for arteriogenic erectile dysfunction: the long-term efficacy calculated by survival analysis." *Br J Urol Int* 94:361–366, 2004.

Kendira M, et al. "The impact of various risk factors on penile hemodynamics in men with ED." Paper presented at the American Urological Association Annual Meeting. Atlanta, GA, May 20–25, 2006.

Kendirci M, et al. "The impact of vascular risk factors on erectile function." *Timely Top Med Cardiovasc Dis* 1:E11, 2005.

Kinsey AC, et al. *Sexual Behavior in the Human Male.* Philadelphia: W. B. Saunders, 1948.

Klotz T, et al. "Why do patients with erectile dysfunction abandon effective therapy with sildenafil (Viagra)?" *Int J Impot Res* 17:2–4, 2005.

Kocakok E, et al. "Effects of sildenafil on major arterial blood flow in duplex sonography." *J Clin Ultrasound* 33:173–175, 2005.

Kostis JB, et al. "Sexual dysfunction and cardiac risk (the Second Princeton Consensus Conference)." *Am J Cardiol* 96:85M–93M, 2005.

Kratzik CW, et al. "Hormone profiles, body mass index and aging male symptoms: results of the Androx Vienna Municipality Study." *Aging Male* 7:188–196, 2004.

Kupelian V, et al. "Erectile dysfunction as a predictor of the metabolic syndrome in aging men: results from the Massachusetts Male Aging Study." *J Urol* 176:222–226, 2006a.

Kupelian V, et al. "The impact of sex hormones on erectile dysfunction: results of the Massachusetts Male Aging Study." Paper presented at the American Urological Association Annual Meeting. Atlanta, GA, May 20–25, 2006b.

Latini DM, et al. "Psychological impact of erectile dysfunction: validation of a new health-related quality-of-life measure for patients with erectile dysfunction." *J Urol* 168:2086–2091, 2002.

Lau DH, et al. "Gene therapy and erectile dysfunction: the current status." *Asian J Androl,* 2008, in press.

Lee PA, Reiter EO. "Genital size: a common adolescent male concern." *Adolesc Med* 13:171–180, 2002.

Lehman K, et al. "Reasons for discontinuing intracavernous injection therapy with prostaglandin E1 (alprostadil)." *Urology* 53:397–400, 1999.

Lepore JJ, et al. "Hemodynamic effects of sildenafil in patients with congestive heart failure and pulmonary hypertension: combined administration with inhaled nitric oxide." *Chest* 127:1647–1653, 2005.

Leslie SJ, et al. "No adverse hemodynamic reaction between sildenafil and red wine." *Clin Pharmacol Ther* 76:365–370, 2004.

Lever J, et al. "Does size matter? Men's and women's views on penis size across life span." *Psychol Men Masculinity* 3:129–143, 2006.

Levine LA, Estrada CR. "Intralesional verapamil for the treatment of Peyronie's disease: a review." *Int J Impot Res* 14:324–328, 2002.

Lewis R, et al. "Epidemiology/risk factors of sexual dysfunction." *J Sex Med* 1:35–39, 2004.

Lizza EF, Rosen RC. "Definition and classification of erectile dysfunction: report of the Nomenclature Committee of the International Society of Impotence Research." *Int J Impot Res* 11:141–143, 1999.

Lobo JR, Nehra A. "Clinical evaluation of erectile dysfunction in era of PDE 5-inhibitors." *Urol Clin North Am* 32:447–455, 2005.

LoPicollo J. "Post-modern sex therapy for erectile failure." *Nord Sexol* 9:205–225, 1991.

Lue TF. "Male sexual dysfunction." In *Smith's General Urology,* pp. 803–805. New York: Lange Medical Books/McGraw-Hill, 2000.

Lue TF. "Adipose tissue derived stem cells and sexual medicine." Paper presented at the Third Biennial Conference of the Pan Arab Society for Sexual Medicine. Dubai, United Arab Emirates, February 8–11, 2007.

Lue TF, Tanagho EA. "Physiology of erection and pharmacological management of impotence." *J Urol* 137:829, 1987.

Lue T, et al. "Physiology of erection." In *Clinical Manual of Sexual Medicine. Sexual Dysfunctions in Men,* pp. 9–18. Paris: Health Publications, 2004a.

Lue TF, et al. "Summary of the recommendations on sexual dysfunctions in men." *J Sex Med* 1:6–23, 2004b.

Lue T, et al. "Intracorporeal pharmacological therapy." In *Clinical Manual of Sexual Medicine. Sexual Dysfunctions in Men,* pp. 39. Paris: Health Publications, 2004c.

Manikandan R, et al. "Evaluation of extracorporeal shock wave therapy in Peyronie's disease." *Urology* 60:795–791, 2002. (Discussion, *Urology* 60: 799–800, 2002.)

Marshall Y. *"The Rise of Viagra: How the Little Blue Pill Changed Sex in America,* by Meika Loe" [Book Review] *N Engl J Med* 351:2776–2777, 2004.

Martinez-Jabaloyas JM, et al. "Testosterone levels in men with erectile dysfunction." *Br J Urol Int* 97:1278–1283, 2006.

Masters WH, Johnson VE. *Human Sexual Inadequacy.* Boston: Little-Brown, 1970.

McMahon CG, Meston C. "Definitions and Epidemiology of Sexual Dysfunction." Paper presented at the Second International Consultation on Erectile and Sexual Dysfunctions. Paris, June 28–July 1, 2003.

McMahon CG, Montorsi F. "Premature ejaculation: past, present, and future perspectives: introduction." Paper presented at the 11th World Congress of the International Society for Sexual and Impotence Research. Buenos Aires, Argentina, October 18–21, 2004.

McMahon CG, et al. "Disorders of orgasm and ejaculation in men." *J Sex Med* 1:58–65, 2004.

McMahon CG, et al. "Efficacy of type-5 phosphodiesterase inhibitors in the drug treatment of premature ejaculation: a systematic review." *Br J Urol Int* 98:259–272, 2006.

McVary KT, et al. "Sildenafil improves erectile function and concomitant lower urinary tract symptoms in men." Paper presented at the American Urological Association Annual Meeting. Atlanta, GA, May 20–25, 2006.

Melman A, et al. "Results of the first human trial for gene transfer therapy for the treatment of erectile dysfunction [Abstract 686]. *J Urol* 175:222, 2006.

Melman A, et al. "Gene transfer with a vector expressing Maxi-K from a smooth muscle specific promoter restores erectile function in the aging rat." *Gene Ther* 15:364–370, 2008.

Metin A, et al. "Does lidocaine ointment addition increase fluoxetine efficacy in the same group of patients with premature ejaculation?" *Urol Int* 75:231–234, 2005.

Meuleman EJH, Van Lankveld JDM. "Hypoactive sexual desire disorder: an underestimated condition in men." *Br J Urol* 95:291–296, 2004.

Meyer KF, et al. "Definitions and epidemiology of sexual dysfunction." Paper presented at the Second International Consultation on Erectile and Sexual Dysfunctions. Paris, June 28–July 1, 2003.

Mikhail N. "Does testosterone have a role in erectile dysfunction?" *Am J Med* 119:372–382, 2006.

Mirone V, et al. "An evaluation of an alternative dosing regimen with tadalafil, 3 time/week for men with erectile dysfunction: SURE study in 14 European countries." *Eur Urol* 47:846–854, 2005.

Mittleman MA, et al. "Evaluation of acute risk for myocardial infarction in men treated with sildenafil citrate." *Am J Cardiol* 96:443–446, 2005.

Mondaini N, Gontero P. "Idiopathic short penis: myth or reality?" *Br J Urol Int* 95:8–10, 2005.

Mondaini N, et al. "Penile size is normal in most men seeking penile lengthening procedures." *Int J Impot Res* 14:283–286, 2002.

Montague DK, et al. "AUA guidelines on the pharmacologic management of premature ejaculation." *J Urol* 172:290–294, 2004.

Montague DK, et al. "Erectile Dysfunction Guideline Update Panel. Chapter 1: The management of erectile dysfunction: an AUA update." *J Urol* 174:230–239, 2005.

Montorsi F. "Peyronie's disease—ESU course, medical and surgical management of erectile dysfunction." Paper presented at the European Association of Urology Meeting. Istanbul, Turkey, March 16–19, 2005.

Montorsi F, et al. "The ageing male and erectile dysfunction." *Br J Urol Int* 92:516–525, 2003.

Montorsi F, et al. "Erectile dysfunction predicts extension of coronary artery disease by angiography in acute coronary syndromes: the dead goose study." Paper presented at the American Urological Association Annual Meeting. Atlanta, GA, May 20–25, 2006.

Morales A. "The andropause: bare facts for urologists." *Br J Urol Int* 91:311–313, 2003.

Morales A. "Testosterone and prostate health: Debunking myths demands evidence, caution and good judgment." *European Urology* 50:895–897, 2006.

Morales A, Heaton JPW. "Hypogonadism and erectile dysfunction: pathophysiological observations and therapeutic outcomes." *Br J Urol Int* 92:896–899, 2003.

Morelli A, et al. "Which patients with sexual dysfunction are suitable for testosterone therapy?" *J Endocrinol Invest* 30:880–888, 2007.

Mueller A, et al. "Analysis of predictors of erectile function outcomes with pharmacological penile rehabilitation following radical prostatectomy." Paper presented at the American Urological Association Annual Meeting. Atlanta, GA, May 20–25, 2006.

Mukhergee B, Shivakumar T. "A case of sensorineural deafness following ingestion of Sildenafil." *J Laryngol Otol* 121:395–397, 2007.

Mykletun A, et al. "Assessment of male sexual function by the Brief Sexual Function Inventory." *Br J Urol Int* 97:316–323, 2006.

Nakanishi S, et al. "Erectile dysfunction is strongly linked with decreased libido in diabetic men." *Aging Male* 7:113–119, 2004.

Padmanabhan P, McCullough AR. "A pilot study to determine local oxygen saturation of the flaccid and erect penis in men with or without erectile dysfunction using a non-invasive tissue oximeter." Paper presented at the American Urological Association Annual Meeting. Atlanta, GA, May 20–25, 2006.

Padma-Nathan H, Yeager JL. "An integrated analysis of alprostadil topical cream for the treatment of erectile dysfunction in 1732 patients." *Urology* 68:386–391, 2006.

Panser LA, et al. "Sexual function of men ages 40 to 79 years: the Olmsted County study of urinary symptoms and health status among men." *J Am Geriatr Soc* 43:1107–1111, 1995.

Patel P. *Sexuality: Perception and Performance throughout History.* Lilly-ICOS, 2006.

Patrick DL, et al. "Premature ejaculation: an observational study of men and their partners." *J Sex Med* 2:358–367, 2005.

Patrick DL, et al. "'He said/she said': comparing male and partner perceptions of premature ejaculation." Paper presented at the American Urological Association Annual Meeting. Atlanta, GA, May 20–25, 2006.

Perelman MA. "Unveiling retarded ejaculation." *J Urol* 175(suppl 4), abstract 1337, 2006.

Perelman M, et al. "Attitudes of men with erectile dysfunction: a cross-national survey." *J Sex Med* 2:397–406, 2005.

Perovic S, et al. "Enlargement and sculpturing of a small and deformed penis." *J Urol* 170:1686–1690, 2003.

Perovic SV, et al. "New perspectives of penile enhancement surgery: tissue engineering with biodegradable scaffolds." *Eur Urol* 49:139–147, 2006.

Pickard RS, et al. "The role of color duplex ultrasonography in the diagnosis of vasculogenic impotence." *Br J Urol* 68:537–540, 1991.

Ponchietti R, et al. "Penile length and circumference: a study of 3,300 Italian males." *Eur Urol* 9:183–186, 2001.

Porst H, et al. "The Premature Ejaculation Prevalence and Attitudes (PEPA) survey: prevalence, comorbidities, and professional help-seeking." *Eur Urol* 26, doi: EUR UROL 51: 816–23, 2007, 2006.

Prins J, et al. "Prevalence of erectile dysfunction: a systematic review of population-based studies." *Int J Impot Res* 14:422–432, 2002.

"Proceedings of the First Latin American Erectile Dysfunction Consensus." *Int J Impot Res* 15(suppl 7):S1–S45, 2003.

Pryor J, et al. "Peyronie's disease." *J Sex Med* 1:110–115, 2004.

Raina R, et al. "Early combination therapy following radical prostatectomy (RP): intracorporeal alprostadil and sildenafil promotes early return of natural erections." Paper presented at the American Urological Association Annual Meeting. Atlanta, GA, May 20–25, 2006.

Rajpurkar A, Dhabuwala CB. "Comparison of satisfaction rates and erectile function in patients treated with sildenafil, intracavernous prostaglandin E1 and penile implant surgery for erectile dysfunction in urology practice." *J Urol* 170:159–163, 2003.

Ralph DJ, Minhas S. "The management of Peyronie's disease." *Br J Urol* 3:208–215, 2004.

Ralph DJ, Wylie KR. "Ejaculatory disorders and sexual function." *Br J Urol* 95:1181–1186, 2005.

Ravipati G, et al. "Type 5 phosphodiesterase inhibitors in the treatment of erectile dysfunction and cardiovascular disease." *Cardiol Rev* 15:76–86, 2007.

Renshaw DC. "Coping with an impotent husband." *Ill Med J* 159:29–35, 1981.

Rivera P, et al. "Use of paroxetine on demand in premature ejaculation." *Actas Urol Esp* 29:387–389, 2005.

Rosano GM, et al. "Chronic treatment with tadalafil improves endothelial function in men with increased cardiovascular risk." *Eur Urol* 47:214–222, 2005.

Rosen R, et al. "Lower urinary tract symptoms and male sexual dysfunction: the Multinational Survey of the Aging Male (MSAM-7)." *Eur Urol* 44:637–649, 2003.

Rosen RC. "Psychogenic erectile dysfunction: classification and management." *Urol Clin N Am* 28:269–278, 2001.

Rosen RC. "Reproductive health problems in ageing men." *Lancet* 366:183–184, 2005.

Rosen RC, et al. "The premature ejaculation prevalence and attitudes (PEPA) survey: a multinational survey." *J Sex Med* 1(suppl):57–58, 2004.

Rosenberg MT, et al. "Premature ejaculation as reported by the female partners: prevalence and sexual satisfaction survey results from a community practice." Paper presented at the American Urological Association Annual Meeting. Atlanta, GA, May 20–25, 2006.

Saad F, et al. "Effects of testosterone gel followed by parenteral testosterone undecanoate on sexual dysfunction and on features of the metabolic syndrome." *Andrologia*
40:44–8, 2008 (in press).

Sadovsky R, Mulhall JP. "The potential value of erectile inquiry and management." *Int J
Clin Pract* 53:601–608, 2003.

Salem EA, et al. "Tramadol HCL has promise in on demand use to treat premature ejaculation." Paper presented at the Third Biennial Conference of the Pan Arab Society for
Sexual Medicine. Dubai, United Arab Emirates, February 8–11, 2007.

Salonia A, et al. "A prospective study comparing paroxetine alone versus paroxetine plus
sildenafil in patients with premature ejaculation." *J Urol* 168:2486–2489, 2002.

Salvi FM. "Au dela d l'orgasm (Beyond orgasm)" [French]. *Pscyhologies* 8:58–61, 2006.

Samraj GPN, et al. "Current and future strategies for premature ejaculation." *Contemp Urol*
17(5):12–21, 2005.

Schaalma HP, et al. "Sex education as health promotion: what does it take?" *Arch Sex Behav*
33:259–269, 2004.

Schneider T, et al. "Does penile size in younger men cause problems in condom use?
A prospective measurement of penile dimensions in 111 young and 32 older men."
Urology 57:314–318, 2001.

Schubert M, Jockenhovel F. "Late onset hypogonadism in the aging male (LOH):
definition, diagnostic and clinical aspects." *J Endocrinol Invest* 28:23–27, 2005.

Schwarz ER, et al. "The effects of chronic phosphodiesterase-5 inhibitor use in different
organ systems." *Int J Impot Res,* 2008, in press.

Seftel A. "Testosterone replacement therapy for male hypogonadism, part III: pharmacologic and clinical profiles, monitoring, safety issues, and potential future agents." *Int
J Impot Res* 19:2–24, 2007.

Seftel AD, et al. "The prevalence of hypertension, hyperlipidemia, diabetes mellitus and
depression in men with erectile dysfunction." *J Urol* 171:2341–2345, 2004.

Seidman SN, Roose SP. "Sexual dysfunction and depression." *Curr Psychiatry Rep*
3:202–208, 2001.

Semans JH. "Premature ejaculation (ejaculation praecox): a new method of therapy." *Z Urol*
52:381–389, 1959.

"Sex education: start discussions early." *Mayo Clinic Newsletter,* June 7, 2005, http://www.
mayoclinic.com.

Shabsigh R, et al. "Drivers and barriers to seeking treatment for erectile dysfunction:
a comparison of six countries." *Br J Urol Int* 94:1055–1065, 2004.

Shabsigh R, et al. "Health issues of men: prevalence and correlates of erectile dysfunction."
J Urol 174:662–667, 2005a.

Shabsigh R, et al. "Time from dosing to sexual intercourse attempts in men taking tadalafil
in clinical trials." *Br J Urol Int* 96:857–863, 2005b.

Sharlip ID. "Course: premature ejaculation." Paper presented at the American Urological
Association Annual Meeting. Atlanta, GA, May 20–25, 2006.

Sighinolfi MC, et al. "Changes in peak systolic velocity induced by chronic therapy with
phosphodiesterase type-5 inhibitor." *Andrologia* 38:84–86, 2006.

Singer AJ. "Management options: clinical applications of the Erectile Dysfunction Guideline 2005 Update Panel." *Issues Urol* 18:85–88, 2006.

Sobel RE, et al. "Nonaeteritic anterior ischemic neuropathy in men using sildenafil citrate
for erectile dysfunction: a review of >44,800 patients in clinical and observational
studies." Paper presented at the American Urological Association Annual Meeting.
Atlanta, GA, May 20–25, 2006.

Sommer F, et al. "Epidemiology of Peyronie's disease." *Int J Impot Res* 14:379–383, 2002.

Sommer F, Schulze W. "Treating erectile dysfunction by endothelial rehabilitation with phosphodiesterase-5 inhibitors." *World J Urol* 23:385–392, 2005.

Son H, et al. "Studies on self-esteem and penile size in young Korean military men." *Asian J Androl* 5:185–189, 2003.

Sotomayar M. "The burden of premature ejaculation: the patient's perspective." *J Sex Med* 2(suppl):110–114, 2005.

Speel TG, et al. "The risk of coronary heart disease in men with erectile dysfunction." *Eur Urol* 44:366–370, 2003. (Discussion, *Eur Urol* 44:370–371, 2003.)

Sultan C, et al. "Disorders linked to insufficient androgen action in male children." *Human Reprod Update* 7:314–322, 2001.

Susman ED. "Vardenafil improves satisfaction among men with premature ejaculation." paper presented at the American Urological Association Annual Meeting. San Antonio, TX, May 23, 2005.

Syropoulos E, et al. "Size of external genital organs and somatometric parameters among physically normal men younger than 40 years old." *Urology* 62:201–204, 2003.

Talalaj J, Talalaj S. *The Strangest Sex: Ceremonies and Customs.* Melbourne, Australia: Hill of Content, 1994.

Thompson IM, et al. "Association of erectile dysfunction and subsequent cardiovascular disease." *J Urol* 175(suppl 4), abstract 1333, 2006.

Tornehl CK, et al. "Peyronie's disease: individualizing the surgical approach." *Contemp Urol* 16(6):34–35, 2004.

Travison TG, et al. "The natural progression and remission of ED: results from the Massachusetts Male Aging Study." *J Urol* 177:241–246, 2007.

Turnbull JM, Weinberg PC. "Psychological factors involved in impotence: a review of the literature." *J Androl* 4:59–66, 1983.

Uckert S. "Update on phosphodiesterase (PDE) isoenzymes as pharmacologic targets in urology: present and future." *Eur Urol,* 2008, in press.

University of South Carolina. "Premature ejaculation: out of the dark ages and into the 21st century." *Urol Times* 33, June 1, 2005 http://www.urologytimes.com.

Vicari E, et al. "Incidence of extragenital vascular disease in patients with erectile dysfunction of arterial origin." *Int J Impot Res* 17:277–282, 2005.

Vignozzi L, et al. "Testosterone and sexual activity." *J Endocrinol Invest* 28:39–44, 2005.

Virag R. "Intracavernous injections and new medical treatments of impotence." *Rev Med Interne* 8(suppl 1):31–35, 1997.

Waknine Y. "Medscape alert: reports of sudden vision loss added to labeling for Viagra, Cialis, Levitra." *Medscape Today,* July 8, 2005, http://www.medscape.com/viewarticle/508112.

Waldinger MD, et al. "Familial occurrence of primary premature ejaculation." *Psychiatr Genet* 8:37–40, 1998.

Waldinger MD, et al. "On-demand SSRI treatment of premature ejaculation: pharmacodynamic limitations for relevant ejaculation delay and subsequent solutions." *J Sex Med* 2:121–131, 2005.

Waldinger MD, Schweitzer DH. "Changing paradigms from a historical DSM-III and DSM-IV view toward an evidence-based definition of premature ejaculation, part III: proposal for DSM-V and UCD-II." *J Sex Med* 3:693–705, 2006.

Webster LJ, et al. "Use of sildenafil for safe improvement of erectile function and quality of life in men with New York Heart Association classes II and III congestive heart failure: a prospective, placebo-controlled, double-blind crossover trial." *Arch Intern Med* 164:514–520, 2004.

Weinsaft JW, et al. "Effects of tadalafil on myocardial blood flow in patients with coronary artery disease." *Coron Artery Dis* 17:493–499, 2006.

Wensing G, et al. "Simultaneous administration of vardenafil and alcohol does not result in a pharmacodynamic or pharmacokinetic interaction in healthy male subjects." *Int J Clin Pharmacol Ther* 44:216–224, 2006.

Wespes E, et al. "Sildenafil non-responders: haemodynamic and morphometric studies." *Eur Urol* 48:136–139, 2005.

Wessells H, et al. "Complications of penile lengthening and augmentation seen at one referral center." *J Urol* 155:1617–1620, 1996a.

Wessells H, et al. "Penile length in the flaccid and erect states: guidelines for penile augmentation." *J Urol* 156:995–997, 1996b.

Whitehead ED, Kyde BJ. "Diabetes-related impotence in the elderly." *Clin Geriatr Med* 6:771–795, 1990.

Wright PJ. "Comparison of phosphodiesterase type 5 (PDE-5) inhibitors." *Int J Clin Pract*, 2008, in press.

Wylie KR. "Treatment outcome of brief couple therapy in psychogenic male erectile disorder." *Arch Sex Behav* 26:527–545, 1997.

Wylie KR, Eardley I. "Penile size and the small penis syndrome." *Br J Urol Int* 99:1449–1455, 2007.

Wyllie MG. "ADAM and the andropause." *Br J Urol Int* 91:883–885, 2003.

Wyllie MG. "Libido and desire: join the club." *Br J Urol Int* 92:323–325, 2005.

Yates AJ, et al. "Sex- and age-related differences in ceramide dihexosides of primary human brain tumors." *Lipids* 34:1–4, 1999.

Young JM, et al. "Tadalafil improved erectile function at twenty-four and thirty-six hours after dosing in men with erectile dysfunction: US trial." *J Androl* 25:310–318, 2005.

Zhang Y, et al. "Sildenafil citrate treatment for erectile dysfunction after kidney transplantation." *Transplant Proc* 37:2100–2103, 2005.

INDEX